MANUAL OF
NURSING
DIAGNOSIS

1993-1994

Including all diagnostic categories approved by the
North American Nursing Diagnosis Association

MARJORY GORDON, PhD, RN, FAAN

Professor of Nursing
Boston College

D0139595

 Mosby

St. Louis Baltimore Boston Chicago London Philadelphia Sydney Toronto

Publisher: Alison Miller
Editor: Terry Van Schaik
Developmental Editor: Janet Livingston
Project Manager: Gayle May Morris
Production Editor: Donna L. Walls
Manufacturing Supervisor: Kathy Grone

SIXTH EDITION
Copyright © 1993 by Mosby–Year Book, Inc.
A Mosby imprint of Mosby–Year Book, Inc.

Previous editions copyrighted 1982, 1985, 1987, 1989, 1991

All rights reserved. No part of this publication may be
reproduced, stored in a retrieval system, or transmitted, in any
form or by any means, electronic, mechanical, photocopying,
recording, or otherwise, without prior written permission from
the publisher.

Permission to photocopy or reproduce solely for internal or
personal use is permitted for libraries or other users registered
with the Copyright Clearance Center, provided that the base fee
of $4.00 per chapter plus $.10 per page is paid directly to the
Copyright Clearance Center, 27 Congress Street, Salem, MA
01970. This consent does not extend to other kinds of copying,
such as copying for general distribution, for advertising or
promotional purposes, for creating new collected works, or for
resale.

Printed in the United States of America

International Standard Book Number 0-8016-6671-6

Mosby–Year Book, Inc.
11830 Westline Industrial Drive
St. Louis, Missouri 63146

93 94 95 96 97 GW/DC 9 8 7 6 5 4 3 2 1

CONTENTS

DIAGNOSTIC CATEGORIES, 51*†

*Diagnoses accepted by the North American Nursing Diagnosis Association appear in boldface type.
†NOTE: If the main treatment for a diagnosis (e.g., drugs or surgery) is outside the scope of nursing practice, the problem is placed under a closely related functional pattern. For example, impaired gas exchange mainly influences the activity-exercise pattern. Syndromes are placed under the pattern corresponding to the causative factor (e.g., disuse or relocation).

PREFACE

This manual provides a quick reference to currently accepted and other nursing diagnoses that provide terms to describe diagnostic judgments. It is useful for learners and expert diagnosticians. Learners will be interested in the concise terms to describe a cluster of signs and symptoms exhibited by the client and guidelines for assessment and diagnosis. Experts can get information quickly by accessing nursing diagnoses in various ways. Each diagnosis is clearly presented on a single page and has an additional blank page for valuable notes about important observations or learning.

Nursing diagnoses are based on a nursing assessment. The use of the functional health pattern typology in the manual provides an easily learned framework for assessment. Diagnoses are grouped under the same functional patterns that also organize the assessment guidelines, documentation format, and the example of documentation. This consistency facilitates the movement from data to diagnosis.

Sample admission assessment guides are included for the individual (adults, infants, and young children), family, and community. Sections on how high-incidence diagnoses can be used to guide assessment and diagnosis and how to use diagnostic categories in other clinical activities (e.g., quality assurance) provide a quick reference. Professional documentation is stressed and diagnosis-based charting is illustrated using the problem-oriented format. A synopsis of legal considerations in the use of diagnoses is included.

This 1993-1994 edition of the *Manual of Nursing Diagnosis* is organized to meet the needs of both novices and expert diagnosticians. Because of interest in the functional health patterns typology and nursing diagnoses, formats and a bibliography on use of functional patterns are included. The increasing use of nursing diagnoses by students and graduate nurses around the world is indicated by the fact that to date the *Manual of Nursing Diagnosis* has been translated into Japanese, Chinese, Swedish, Finnish, and French. It is hoped that this sixth edition will be equally well received both in North American and throughout the world of professional nursing practice.

Marjory Gordon

ACKNOWLEDGMENTS

Diagnostic categories contained in this Manual (except those on shaded pages) are based on the work of the North American Nursing Diagnosis Association.* Diagnostic categories on shaded pages are not currently accepted for clinical testing by the Association but have proved useful in care planning.

*Kim MJ, Moritz DA, editors: *Classification of nursing diagnoses: Proceedings of the Third and Fourth National Conferences (1978, 1980)*, New York, 1982, McGraw-Hill; Kim MJ, McFarland G, McLane A, editors: *Classification of nursing diagnoses: Proceedings of the Fifth National Conference (1982)*, St. Louis, 1984, Mosby–Year Book; Hurley M, editor: *Classification of nursing diagnoses: Proceedings of the Sixth Conference (1984)*, St. Louis, 1986, Mosby–Year Book; McLane A, editor: *Classification of nursing diagnoses: Proceedings of the Seventh Conference (1986)*, St. Louis, 1987, Mosby–Year Book; Carroll-Johnson R, editor: *Classification of nursing diagnoses: Proceedings of the Eighth Conference (1988)*, Philadelphia, 1989, Lippincott; North American Nursing Diagnosis Association: *Taxonomy I*, Revised, 1990; 1992; the diagnosis of parent-infant separation was suggested to the author by T. Heather Herdman, Doctoral Student, Boston College School of Nursing.

USE OF THE MANUAL

A diagnostic manual can serve multiple purposes. For students, it is a quick reference during clinical practice, a useful guide in class or clinical conference, and a necessity for doing homework. For expert diagnosticians, it is a clinical reference, a research tool, a teaching or management resource, and a stimulus for ideas. For both learners and experts, it is a much used companion.

This manual contains the most up-to-date diagnostic categories accepted by the North American Nursing Diagnosis Association (NANDA) and contained in NANDA Taxonomy I (Revised 1990) endorsed by the American Nurses Association. It has six main uses that can facilitate the nursing diagnosis-based component of practice:

1. **Access to Diagnoses.** It is a quick reference to terms used in formulating nursing diagnoses.
2. **Functional Health Pattern Assessment and Diagnosis.** Guides are included for linking assessment and diagnosis using functional health patterns and diagnostic groupings.
3. **Diagnosis-Specific Treatment.** Formats for diagnosis-specific treatment plans are outlined.
4. **Documentation.** Format, guidelines, and examples of documentation are provided.
5. **Special Notes.** Pages are included for special notes on specific nursing diagnoses.
6. **Prevention of Harm: The Legal Aspects.** Discussion of legal considerations in nursing diagnosis.

Using this manual for each of these purposes is discussed below.

ACCESS TO DIAGNOSES

Different situations require different ways of accessing nursing diagnoses. The manual can accommodate the following needs:

1. To find a diagnostic category to describe a cluster of signs and symptoms within a functional pattern area, use the Contents (pages iv–ix). Diagnoses are grouped by functional patterns, and each diagnosis is clearly presented on its own page.
2. When a diagnostic category label is known but you need to check the definition, defining characteristics, or etiological/related factors, use the Alphabetical Index to look up the page number. The Alphabetical Index serves as a dictionary of diagnostic terms (pages 357–365).
3. If you wish to scan all the pages of diagnostic categories within a particular functional pattern area, use the Contents (pages iv–ix).

For research on NANDA-accepted diagnostic categories and the taxonomy, use diagnostic categories in R Carroll-Johnson's *Classification of Nursing Diagnoses: Proceedings of the Tenth Conference on Classification of Nursing Diagnoses* (Philadelphia, 1993, Lippincott) and the North American Nursing Diagnosis Association's *Taxonomy I, Revised* (1992).

The diagnostic categories contained in this manual are concepts used in thinking, and they represent a language for communicating. They are used to describe professional nurses' diagnostic judgments about actual or potential health problems and health-related conditions. A useful nursing diagnosis statement consists of terms describing (1) the individual's, the family's, or

the community's health problem/condition and (2) the primary
etiological or related factor(s) contributing to the problem/condi-
tion that is the focus of nursing treatment. In many instances the
client's problem can be formulated by using one diagnostic category to describe the problem and another category from the
same, or a different functional pattern area, to describe etiological factors.

Many types of judgments are made in practice, but the term
nursing diagnosis is reserved for client conditions "which nurses
by virtue of their education and experience are capable and li-
censed to treat" (Gordon, 1976, p. 1299). The North American
Nursing Diagnosis Association's definition of a nursing diagnosis
further clarifies the term:

A nursing diagnosis is a clinical judgment about an individual, family, or
community response to actual or high risk health problems/life processes
which provides the basis for definitive therapy toward achievment of outcomes for which the nurse is accountable (NANDA, 1990).

This builds on a definition based on Shoemaker's research,
which integrates nursing diagnosis into nursing process:

Nursing diagnosis is a clinical judgment about an individual, family, or
community that is derived through a deliberate, systematic process of data
collection and analysis. It provides the basis for prescriptions for definitive
therapy for which the nurse is accountable. It is expressed concisely and
includes the etiology of the condition when known (Shoemaker, 1984, p.
109).

An additional characteristic that distinguishes nursing diagnoses
is that professional nurses assume responsibility for research on
the conditions, their treatment, and outcomes. Nursing diagnoses
are conditions primarily resolved by nursing care methods, and
nurses assume accountability in practice for treatment outcomes.
If a diagnosis does not meet these criteria, a notation to refer the

problem for medical evaluation will be found on the page containing the diagnosis.

Nurses view the diagnostic categories in this manual from various conceptual perspectives. Depending on the model of nursing used to guide the nursing process, diagnoses may be viewed as ineffective adaptations, self-care agency deficits, human response patterns, needs, or, simply, dysfunctional health patterns. There is no consensus on the conceptual focus of nursing and thus no consensus on the focus of nursing diagnosis.

Users of the manual should recognize that nursing diagnoses are in the process of development. In a few diagnostic categories, definitions and labels have been made more concise, defining characteristics reordered for ease of use, and etiological or related factors added or modified. *A few diagnostic categories found to be useful in clinical practice but not yet accepted are included on shaded pages.*

Diagnostic categories require conceptual work and further clinical testing. It is expected that nurses will modify, delete, and add to the currently accepted classifications. Revisions will occur as diagnoses are used (1) to organize assessment data, (2) as a basis for care planning, and (3) as a focus for nursing documentation. Nurses are encouraged to submit refinements of accepted diagnoses to the North American Nursing Diagnosis Association, St. Louis University School of Nursing, 3525 Caroline St., St. Louis, MO 63104.

All diagnostic categories describing problems contain the following components: diagnostic category label, definition, defining characteristics, and etiological or related factors. *An asterisk denotes critical, or major, defining characteristics.* In the opinion of the developers, these are the characteristics that must be present when the label is used. High-risk (potential) problems have risk factors instead of defining characteristics and etiological factors. Healthy states or processes have supporting factors rather than etiological/related factors on which interventions are based (e.g., effective breastfeeding).

FUNCTIONAL HEALTH PATTERN ASSESSMENT AND DIAGNOSIS

The manual contains an assessment format and diagnostic groupings that facilitate the move from data to diagnosis. Both employ the functional health patterns as a nursing perspective on individual, family, and community health care. It is possible that cognitive strain and diagnostic errors can be reduced if there is consistency between organization of assessment data and grouping of diagnostic categories. For example, if data on the client's elimination pattern can be compared to defining characteristics of diagnoses in the elimination pattern, less effort is required than when using an unorganized data base and over 100 alphabetized diagnoses. The following are guidelines for use of the manual in the diagnostic phase of nursing process:

1. Use the manual both to learn the eleven functional health patterns typology and to study the diagnostic categories commonly occurring in your practice area. Functional patterns are an easily learned nursing model for assessment. Review the diagram on Components of Nursing Process, pages 34-35, to place nursing diagnosis in the context of nursing process/clinical judgment.

2. Use the assessment guidelines (pages 9-32) that are based on the functional health pattern areas (pages 2-5) to collect and organize a nursing history/examination of adults (pages 10-15), infants and young children (pages 15-20), families (pages 20-24), or communities (pages 24-30). Also contained in the manual is a bibliography of articles on the use of functional health patterns in clinical activities (page 5-7).

3. If assessment reveals a dysfunctional pattern but the name escapes you, check the diagnoses listed under the pattern (Contents, pages iv-ix) for terminology to label the condition. Use the defining characteristics listed with each diagnosis to validate your judgment. Etiological or risk factors listed with each diagnosis may suggest possible reasons for the problem or high risk state.

4. For a quick reference before documenting a problem, use either the Contents (pages iv-ix), the Alphabetical Index (end pages), or the page numbers for functional pattern areas (outside back cover). Turn to the page corresponding to the possible diagnostic label. Check that observed signs and symptoms correspond to defining characteristics of the diagnostic category.

DIAGNOSIS-SPECIFIC TREATMENT

The nursing diagnosis is used as a basis for projecting outcomes, planning interventions, and evaluating outcome attainment. The problem statement is the basis for outcome projection, that is, the identification of behaviors that signify resolution of the problem. These projected outcomes are then used to document progress toward outcome attainment and to evaluate resolution of the problem.

The etiological factor(s) are the focus for designing interventions that will reduce or eliminate the factors contributing to the problem (see McCloskey & Bulechek, 1992). Outcome attainment is the measure of effectiveness of the intervention. In the case of a potential problem, reduction or elimination of risk factors is the desired outcome.

DOCUMENTATION

The Recording Format Guidelines and Checkpoints (pages 39-41) will be useful in assuring consistency between the nursing diagnosis, the projected outcome, and the intervention plan. An example is provided (pages 45-49).

Documentation is important for statistical purposes. Currently a nursing minimum data set (NMDS) is being studied. This requires documentation of nursing diagnoses, interventions, and outcomes. It will also include an acuity factor (Werley & Lang, 1988).

SPECIAL NOTES

It is important to learn from practice, rather than just practicing. One of the ways to continue learning is to develop the habit of reflecting on insights and new information, creative interventions, or cost-effective methods. Pages labeled "NOTES" are valuable for recording clinical information related to each diagnosis such as important additional cues or etiological factors that have been observed, factors related to a specific population of clients, and interventions that are successful in reaching projected outcomes.

Gordon M: Nursing diagnosis and the diagnostic process, *Am J Nurs* 76:1276-1300, 1976.

McCloskey J, Bulechek GM: *Nursing interventions classification (NIC)*, St. Louis, 1992, Mosby–Year Book.

Shoemaker J: Essential features of a nursing diagnosis. In Kim MJ, McFarland G, McLane A, editors: *Classification of nursing diagnoses: Proceedings of the Fifth National Conference*, St. Louis, 1984, Mosby–Year Book.

Werley H, Lang N: *Identification of the nursing minimum data set*, New York, 1988, Springer.

FUNCTIONAL HEALTH
PATTERNS TYPOLOGY

This section contains (1) definitions of health patterns used for organizing assessment and grouping nursing diagnoses, (2) assessment guidelines based on the definitions, and (3) a documentation format and example.

TYPOLOGY

Functional health patterns of clients, whether individuals, families, or communities, evolve from client-environment interaction. Each pattern is an expression of biopsychosocial integration. No one pattern can be understood without knowledge of the other patterns. Functional patterns are influenced by biological, developmental, cultural, social, and spiritual factors. Dysfunctional health patterns (described by nursing diagnoses) may occur with disease; dysfunctional health patterns also may lead to disease.

The judgment of whether a pattern is functional or dysfunctional is made by comparing assessment data to one or more of the following: (1) individual baselines, (2) established norms for age groups, (3) cultural, social, or other norms. A particular pattern has to be evaluated in the context of other patterns and its contribution to optimal function of the client assessed.

1 HEALTH-PERCEPTION-HEALTH-MANAGEMENT PATTERN

Describes the client's perceived pattern of health and well-being and how health is managed. Includes the individual's perception of health status and its relevance to current activities and future planning. Also included is the individual's health risk management and general health care behavior, such as adherence to mental and physical health promotion activities, medical or nursing prescriptions, and follow-up care.

2 NUTRITIONAL-METABOLIC PATTERN

Describes pattern of food and fluid consumption relative to metabolic need and pattern indicators of local nutrient supply. Includes the individual's patterns of food and fluid consumption: daily eating times, the types and quantity of food and fluids consumed, particular food preferences, and the use of nutrient or vitamin supplements. Describes breastfeeding and infant feeding patterns. Includes reports of any skin lesions and general ability to heal. The condition of skin, hair, nails, mucous membranes, and teeth, and measures of body temperature, height, and weight are included.

3 ELIMINATION PATTERN

Describes patterns of excretory function (bowel, bladder, and skin). Includes the individual's perceived regularity of excretory function, use of routines or laxatives for bowel elimination, and any changes or disturbances in time-pattern, mode of excretion, quality, or quantity. Also included are any devices employed to control excretion.

4 ACTIVITY-EXERCISE PATTERN

Describes pattern of exercise, activity, leisure, and recreation. Includes activities of daily living requiring energy expenditure, such as hygiene, cooking, shopping, eating, working, and home maintenance. Also included are the type, quantity, and quality of exercise, including sports, which describe the typical pattern for the individual. Factors that interfere with the desired or expected pattern for the individual (such as neuromuscular deficits and compensations, dyspnea, angina, or muscle cramping on exertion, and cardiac/pulmonary classification, if appropriate) are included. Leisure patterns are also included and describe the activities the individual undertakes as recreation either with a group or as an individual. Emphasis is on the activities of high importance or significance to the individual.

5 SLEEP-REST PATTERN

Describes patterns of sleep, rest, and relaxation. Includes patterns of sleep and rest-relaxation periods during the 24-hour day. Includes the individual's perception of the quality and quantity of sleep and rest, and perception of energy level. Included also are aids to sleep such as medications or nighttime routines that the individual employs.

6 COGNITIVE-PERCEPTUAL PATTERN

Describes sensory-perceptual and cognitive pattern. Includes the adequacy of sensory modes, such as vision, hearing, taste, touch, or smell, and the compensation or prothesthetics utilized for disturbances. Reports of pain perception and how pain is managed are also included when appropriate. Also included are the cognitive functional abilities, such as language, memory, and decision making.

7 SELF-PERCEPTION–SELF-CONCEPT PATTERN

Describes self-concept pattern and perceptions of self. Includes the individual's attitudes about himself or herself, perception of abilities (cognitive, affective, or physical), body image, identity, general sense of worth, and general emotional pattern. Pattern of body posture and movement, eye contact, voice, and speech pattern are included.

8 ROLE-RELATIONSHIP PATTERN

Describes pattern of role engagements and relationships. Includes the individual's perception of the major roles and responsibilities in current life situation. Satisfaction or disturbances in family, work, or social relationships and responsibilities related to these roles are included.

9 SEXUALITY-REPRODUCTIVE PATTERN

Describes patterns of satisfaction or dissatisfaction with sexuality; describes reproductive pattern. Includes the individual's perceived satisfaction or disturbances in his or her sexuality. Included also is the female's reproductive stage, pre- or postmenopause, and any perceived problems.

10 COPING–STRESS-TOLERANCE PATTERN

Describes general coping pattern and effectiveness of the pattern in terms of stress tolerance. Includes the individual's reserve or capacity to resist challenge to self-integrity, modes of handling stress, family or other support systems, and perceived ability to control and manage situations.

11 VALUE-BELIEF PATTERN

Describes patterns of values, goals, or beliefs (including spiritual) that guide choices or decisions. Includes what is perceived as important in life, quality of life, and any perceived conflicts in values, beliefs, or expectations that are health related.

BIBLIOGRAPHY:

The following references describe functional health patterns, suggested uses of the patterns, and reports of clinical use and research.

Beyea S, Matzo M: Assessing elders using the functional health pattern assessment model, *Nurse Educ* 14:32-37, 1989.
Bryant SO, Kopeski LM: Psychiatric nursing assessment of the eating disorder client, *Top Clin Nurs* 8:57-66, 1986.
Burns C: Development and content validity testing of a comprehensive classifi-

cation of diagnoses for pediatric nurse practitioners, *Nurs Diagn* 2:93-104, 1991.

Burns C: *Development and field testing of a classification of diagnoses for use by pediatric nurse practitioners*, doctoral dissertation, Eugene, 1989, University of Oregon.

Coler MS, Vincent KG: Coded nursing diagnoses on axes: A prioritized, computer-ready diagnostic system for psychiatric-mental health nurses, *Arch Psychiatr Nurs* 1:125-131, 1987.

Collard A, Jones DA, Fitzmaurice J. In McLane A, editor: *Classification of nursing diagnoses: Proceedings of the Seventh Conference*, St. Louis, 1987, Mosby–Year Book, pp. 283-289.

Corrigan JO. Functional health pattern assessment in the emergency department, *J Emerg Nurs* 12:163-167, 1986.

Decker SD, Knight L: Functional health pattern assessment: A seasonal farm-worker community, *J Community Health Nurs* 7:141-151, 1990.

Di Blasi M, Savage J: Revitalizing a documentation system, *Rehabil Nurs* 17:27-9, 1992.

Dion P, Fitzmaurice J, Baer C: Organization of patient assessment data and nursing diagnosis. In McLane A, editor: *Classification of nursing diagnoses: Proceedings of the Seventh Conference*, St. Louis, 1987, Mosby–Year Book, pp. 169-173.

Doyer B, Macker N, Radovich H: Functional health patterns: A post-anesthesia care unit's approach to identification, *J Post Anesth Nurs* 5:157-162, 1990.

Gilmartin ME: Patient and family education, *Clin Chest Med* 7:619-627, 1986.

Gordon M: *Nursing diagnosis: Process and application*, New York, 1987, McGraw-Hill, pp. 91-161.

Gordon M: Practice-based data set for a nursing information system, *J Med Systems* 9:43-55, 1985.

Greenlee KK: Effects of implementation of an operational definition and guidelines for the formulation of nursing diagnoses in a critical care setting. In Carroll-Johnson R, editor: *Classification of nursing diagnoses: Proceedings of the Ninth Conference*, St Louis, 1991, Mosby–Year Book, pp. 274-275.

Hanna D, Wyman N: Assessment + diagnosis = care planning: A tool for co-ordination, *Nurs Manage* 18:106-109, 1989.

Hartman D, Knudson J: Documentation: A nursing data base for initial patient assessment, *Oncol Nurs Forum* 18:125-130, 1991.

Henning M: Comparison of nursing diagnostic statements using a functional health pattern and health history/body systems format. In Carroll-Johnson R, editor: *Classification of nursing diagnoses: Proceedings of the Ninth Conference*, St Louis, 1991, Mosby–Year Book, pp. 278-279.

Herberth L, Gosnell DJ: Nursing diagnosis for oncology nursing practice, *Cancer Nurs* 10:41-51, 1987.

Hirschfield-Bartek J, Dow KH: Decreasing documentation time using a patient self-assessment tool, *Oncol Nurs Forum* 17:251-255, 1990.

Leahy MK: Using nursing diagnosis as an organizing framework in an inter-grated curriculum. In *From theory to practice: Abstracts of the Second Nursing Theory Congress*, Toronto, Ontario, 1988, p. 65. (Address: M. Leahy, Instructor of Nursing, Boise State University, Boise, Idaho.)

Levin RF, Crosley JM: Focused data collection for the generation of nursing diagnoses, *J Nurs Staff Dev* 4:56-64, 1986.

Mumma CM, editor: *Rehabilitation nursing: Concepts and practice—a core curriculum,* ed 2, Evanston, IL, 1987, Rehabilitation Nursing Foundation.

Mc Farland G, Thomas MD: *Psychiatric mental health nursing,* Philadelphia, 1990, Lippincott.

Nettle C, Jones N, Pifer P: Community nursing diagnoses, *Commun Health Nurs* 6:135-145, 1989.

Phelan C, Finnell MD, Mottla KA: A patient self-assessment tool for cardiac rehabilitation, *Rehabil Nurs* 14:81, 84-7, 1989.

Rantz M, Miller TV: How diagnoses are changing in long term care, *Am J Nurs* 87:360-361, 1987.

Rossi L: Organizing data for nursing diagnosis using functional health patterns. In McLane A, editor: *Classification of nursing diagnoses: Proceedings of the Seventh Conference,* St Louis, 1987, Mosby–Year Book, pp. 97-102.

Tompkins ES: In support of the discipline of nursing: A nursing assessment, *Nurs Connect* 2:21-29, 1989.

Ward CR: Proportion of specific agreement as a measure of intrarater reliability in the diagnostic process. In McLane A, editor: *Classification of nursing diagnoses: Proceedings of the Seventh Conference,* St Louis, 1987, Mosby–Year Book, pp. 169-173.

Westwell J, et al: Health patterns assessment: A form designed to allow psychiatric nurses to practice theoretical pluralism. In *From Theory to Practice. Abstracts of the Second Nursing Theory Congress,* Toronto, Ontario, 1988.

Woodtli MA, Van Ort S: Nursing diagnoses and functional health patterns in patients receiving external radiation therapy: Cancer of the head and neck, *Nurs Diagn* 2:171-180, 1991.

FUNCTIONAL HEALTH PATTERNS ASSESSMENT GUIDELINES

Functional health patterns provide a format for the admission assessment and a data base for nursing diagnosis. There are two phases in assessment: history taking and examination. A nursing history provides a description of a client's functional patterns. The description is from the individual's (or parent's/guardian's), family's, or community representative's perspective and provides data in the form of verbal reports. These are elicited by questions. Observations in the examination phase provide data on pattern indicators and verification of information obtained during history taking.

The formats for assessment that follow are designed to elicit information in a systematic manner. They are screening formats for the collection of a basic nursing data base in any specialty, for any age group, and at any point in the wellness-illness continuum. If data indicate that a problem or potential problem (dysfunctional pattern) may be present, diagnostic hypotheses should be generated to direct further information collection.

Nurses practicing in a specialty area may wish detailed assessments of certain patterns. Both the history (subjective data) and the examination (objective data) can be expanded relative to disease, disability, age, and other client-specific factors. For example, a client's activity-exercise pattern requires an in-depth assessment when the client has a disease that impacts on this pattern.

Diagnoses are grouped under the same pattern areas as in the assessment guidelines and can be used to label data in a pattern area. As discussed previously, this facilitates the process of moving from assessment to diagnosis.

ADULT ASSESSMENT

NURSING HISTORY

1. *Health-perception–health-management pattern*
   a. How has general health been?

   b. Any colds in past year? If appropriate, absences from work/school?

   c. Most important things do to keep healthy? Think these things make a difference to health? (Include family folk remedies, if appropriate). Breast self-examination? Use cigarettes? Drugs? Ever had a drinking problem? When was your last drink?

   d. Accidents (home, work, driving)?

   e. In past, been easy to find ways to follow things doctors or nurses suggest?

   f. If appropriate: What do you think caused this illness? Action taken when symptoms perceived? Results of action?

   g. If appropriate: Things important to you while you're here? How can we be most helpful?

2. *Nutritional-metabolic pattern*

   a. Typical daily food intake? (Describe.) Supplements?

   b. Typical daily fluid intake? (Describe.)

   c. Weight loss/gain? (Amount) Height loss/gain? (Amount)

   d. Appetite?

   e. Food or eating: Discomfort? Swallowing? Diet restrictions? If appropriate: Breastfeeding? Problems?

   f. Heal well or poorly?

   g. Skin problems: Lesions, dryness?

   h. Dental problems?

3. *Elimination pattern*

   a. Bowel elimination pattern. (Describe.) Frequency? Character? Discomfort? Problem in control? Laxatives?

   b. Urinary elimination pattern. (Describe.) Frequency? Problem in control?

   c. Excess perspiration? Odor problems?

4. *Activity-exercise pattern*

   a. Sufficient energy for desired/required activities?

    b. Exercise pattern? Type? Regularity?

    c. Spare time (leisure) activities? Child: Play activities?

    d. Perceived ability for: (code for level)

Feeding _____	Grooming _____
Bathing _____	General mobility _____
Toileting _____	Cooking _____
Bed mobility _____	Home maintenance _____
Dressing _____	Shopping _____

    Functional Levels Code

    Level 0:   Full self-care

    Level I: Requires use of equipment or device

    Level II: Requires assistance or supervision from another person

    Level III: Requires assistance or supervision from another person and equipment or device

    Level IV: Is dependent and does not participate

5. *Sleep-rest pattern*

    a. Generally rested and ready for daily activities after sleep?

    b. Sleep onset problems? Aids? Dreams (nightmares)? Early awakening?

    c. Rest/relaxation periods?

6. *Cognitive-perceptual pattern*

    a. Hearing difficulty? Aid?

    b. Vision? Wear glasses? Last checked?

    c. Any change in memory lately?

    d. Easy/difficult to make decisions?

    e. Easiest way for you to learn things? Any difficulty learning?

    f. Any discomfort? Pain? How do you manage it?

7. *Self-perception–self-concept pattern*

    a. How would you describe yourself? Most of the time, feel good (not so good) about yourself?

    b. Changes in your body or the things you can do? Problem to you?

      c. Changes in way you feel about yourself or your body (since illness started)?

      d. Find things frequently make you angry? Annoyed? Fearful? Anxious? Depressed? What helps?

      e. Ever feel you lose hope? Not able to control things in life? What helps?

8. *Role-relationship pattern*

      a. Live alone? Family? Family structure (diagram)?

      b. Any family problems you have difficulty handling? (nuclear/extended)

      c. How does family usually handle problems?

      d. Family depend on you for things? How managing?

      e. If appropriate: How family/others feel about your illness/hospitalization?

      f. If appropriate: Problems with children? Difficulty handling?

      g. Belong to social groups? Close friends? Feel lonely (frequency)?

      h. Things generally go well for you at work? (School?) If appropriate: Income sufficient for needs?

      i. Feel part of (or isolated in) neighborhood where living?

9. *Sexuality-reproductive pattern*

      a. If appropriate to age/situation: Sexual relationships satisfying? Changes? Problems?

      b. If appropriate: Use of contraceptives? Problems?

      c. Female: When menstruation started? Last menstrual period? Menstrual problems? Para? Gravida?

10. *Coping–stress-tolerance pattern*

      a. Any big changes in your life in the last year or two? Crisis?

      b. Who's most helpful in talking things over? Available to you now?

      c. Tense a lot of the time? What helps? Use any medicines, drugs, alcohol?

   d. When (if) have big problems (any problems) in your
      life, how do you handle them?
   e. Most of the time, is this (are these) way(s) success-
      ful?
11. *Value-belief pattern*
   a. Generally get things you want out of life? Important
      plans for the future?
   b. Religion important in your life? If appropriate: Does
      this help when difficulties arise?
   c. If appropriate: Will being here interfere with any reli-
      gious practices?
12. *Other*
   a. Any other things that we haven't talked about that
      you'd like to mention?
   b. Questions?

SCREENING EXAMINATION FORMAT

(May add other pattern indicators to expand the examination)
General appearance, grooming, hygiene _____
Oral mucous membranes (color, moistness, lesions) _____
Teeth: Dentures _____ Cavities _____ Missing _____
Hears whisper? _____
Reads newsprint? _____ Glasses? _____
Pulse (rate) _____ (rhythm) _____ (strength) _____
Respiration ___ (depth) ___ (rhythm) ___ Breath sounds ___
Blood pressure _____
Hand grip _____ Can pick up pencil? _____
Range of motion (joints) _____ Muscle firmness _____
Skin: Bony prominences ___ Lesions ___ Color changes ___
Gait _____ Posture _____ Absent body part _____
Demonstrated ability for: (Code for Level)
Feeding _____   Grooming _____
Bathing _____   General mobility _____
Toileting _____   Cooking _____

Bed mobility _____   Home maintenance _____
Dressing _____   Shopping _____
Intravenous, drainage, suction, etc. (specify) _____
Actual weight _____ Reported weight _____
Height _____ Temperature _____
During history and examination:
Orientation _____ Grasp Ideas and Questions (abstract,
concrete)? _____
Language spoken _____ Voice and speech pattern _____
Vocabulary Level _____
Eye contact _____ Attention span (distraction) _____
Nervous or relaxed (rate from 1 to 5) _____
Assertive or passive (rate from 1 to 5) _____
Interaction with family member, guardian, other (if
present) _____

INFANT AND YOUNG CHILD ASSESSMENT:

When a new infant or child is added to a nurse's caseload, a
comprehensive assessment is done to establish a data base for
developmental assessment and for nursing diagnosis and treatment. Information is needed on (1) the development of each
functional pattern/anatomical growth, (2) current health patterns,
and (3) family health/home environment in which the infant/
child is developing. Minimally, the admission nursing history/
examination has to screen for high-incidence problems. The
questions/items listed below can be used as a guide for a comprehensive parent-child health history or used selectively for
problem screening.

NURSING HISTORY

1. *Health-perception–health-management pattern*
   Parents' report of:
   a. Mother's pregnancy/labor/delivery history (of this
      infant, of others)?

   b. Infant's health status since birth?
   c. Adherence to routine health checks for the infant/child? Immunizations?
   d. Infections in the infant/child? Child's absences from school?
   e. If applicable: Infant's/child's medical problem, treatment, and prognosis?
   f. If applicable: Actions taken by parents when signs/symptoms perceived?
   g. If appropriate: Has it been easy to follow doctors' or nurses' suggestions?
   h. Preventive health practices (e.g., diaper change, utensils, and clothes)?
   i. Do parents smoke? Around children?
   j. Accidents? Frequency?
   k. Infant's crib toys (safety)? Carrying safety? Car safety?
   l. Parents' safety practices (e.g., household products, and medicines)
   Parents (self):
   a. Parents'/family's general health status?

2. *Nutritional-metabolic pattern*
   Parents' report of the infant's/child's:
   a. Breast/bottle feeding? Intake (estimated)? Sucking strength?
   b. Appetite? Feeding discomfort?
   c. Twenty-four-hour intake of nutrients? Supplements?
   d. Eating behavior? Food preferences? Conflicts over food?
   e. Birth weight? Current weight?
   f. Skin problems: Rashes, lesions, etc.?
   Parents (self):
   a. Parents'/family's nutritional status? Problems?

3. *Elimination pattern*

Parents' report of the infant's/child's:

   a. Bowel elimination pattern? (Describe.) Frequency? Character discomfort?

   b. Diaper changes? (Describe routine.)

   c. Urinary elimination pattern? (Describe.) Number of wet diapers per day? (Estimate amount.) Stream (strong, dribble)?

   d. Excess perspiration? Odor?

Parents (self):

   a. Elimination pattern? Problems?

4. *Activity-exercise pattern*

Parents' report of:

   a. Bathing routine? (When, how, where, and what type of soap?)

   b. Dressing routine? (Clothing worn, changes inside/outside home)

   c. Typical day's activity for the infant/child (hours spent in crib, being carried, playing, etc.; type of toys used)?

   d. Infant's/child's general activity level? Tolerance?

   e. Perception of infant's/child's strength (*strong* or *fragile*)?

   f. Child's self-care ability (bathing, feeding, toileting, dressing, grooming)?

Parents (self):

   a. Activity/exercise/leisure pattern? Child care? Home maintenance?

5. *Sleep-rest pattern*

Parents' report of:

   a. Sleep pattern of the infant/child: Estimated hours?

   b. Infant's/child's restlessness? Nightmares? Nocturia?

   c. Infant's sleep position? Body movements?

Parents (self):

a. Sleep pattern?

6. *Cognitive-perceptual pattern*

Parents' report of:

a. General responsiveness of the infant/child?

b. Infant's response to talking? Noise? Objects? Touch?

c. Infant's following of objects with eyes? Response to crib toys?

d. Learning (changes noted)? What is being taught to the infant/child?

e. Noises/vocalizations? Speech pattern? Words? Sentences?

f. Use of stimulation: Talking, games, etc.?

g. Vision, hearing, touch, kinesthesia of the infant/ child?

h. Child's ability to tell name, time, address, telephone number?

i. Infant's/child's ability to identify needs (hunger, thirst, pain, discomfort)?

Parents (self):

a. Problems with vision, hearing, touch, etc.?

b. Difficulties making decisions? Judgments?

7. *Self-perception–self-concept pattern*

Parent's report of:

a. Infant's/child's mood state (irritability)?

b. Child's sense of worth, identity, competency?

Child's report of:

a. Mood state?

b. Many/few friends? Liked by others?

c. Self-perception ("good" most of time? Hard to be "good"?)

d. Ever lonely?

e. Fears (transient/frequent)?

Parents (self):

a. General sense of worth, identity, competency?

b. Self-perception as parents?

8. *Role-relationship pattern*

Parent's report of:

a. Family/household structure?

b. Family problems/stressors?

c. Interactions among family members and infant (or child)?

d. Infant's/child's response to separation?

e. Child: Dependency?

f. Child: Play pattern?

g. Child: Temper tantrums? Discipline problems? School adjustment?

Parents (self):

a. Role engagements? Satisfaction?

b. Work/social/marital relationships?

9. *Sexuality–reproductive pattern*

Parents' report of child's:

a. Feeling of maleness/femaleness?

b. Questions regarding sexuality? How parent responds?

Parents (self):

a. If applicable: Reproductive history?

b. Sexual satisfaction/problems?

10. *Coping–stress-tolerance pattern*

Parents' report of:

a. What produces stress in child? Level of stress toler-ance?

b. Child's pattern of handling problems, frustrations, an-ger, etc.?

Parents (self):

a. Life stressors? Family stress?

b. Strategies for handling problems? Support systems?

11. *Value-belief pattern*
   Parents' report of:
   a. Child's moral development, choice behavior, commit-
      ments?
   Parents (self):
   a. Things important in life (values, spirituality)? Desires
      for the future?
   b. If appropriate: Perceived impact of disease on goals?

12. *Other*
   a. Any other things that we haven't talked about that
      you'd like to mention? Any questions?

SCREENING EXAMINATION FORMAT

a. General appearance of infant/child _____
b. General appearance of parent(s) _____
c. Child's height/weight _____ Structural growth and development _____
d. Skin color, hydration, rashes, lesions _____
e. If warranted: Child's/Infant's urine and stool _____
f. Reflexes (appropriate to age) _____
   Blood pressure _____
g. Breathing pattern; rate, rhythm _____
h. Heart sounds; rate, rhythm _____
i. Infant/child: Responsiveness, cognitive-perceptual development _____
j. Child: Eye contact, speech pattern, posturing _____
k. Smiling response (infant) _____
l. Social interaction (child)? Aggressive/withdrawn? _____
m. Response to vocalizations? Requests? _____

FAMILY ASSESSMENT

   The 11 functional health pattern areas are applicable to the
assessment of families. Families are the primary client in com-

munity health nursing. In some cases a family assessment may be indicated (1) in the care of an infant or child whose development is influenced by family health patterns or (2) when an adult has certain health problems that can be influenced by family patterns. The following guidelines provide information on family functioning:

1. *Health-perception–health-management pattern*
   History:
   a. How has family's general health been (in last few years)?
   b. Colds in past year? Absence from work/school?
   c. Most important things you do to keep healthy? Think these make a difference to health? (Include family folk remedies, if appropriate.)
   d. Members' use of cigarettes, alcohol, drugs?
   e. Immunizations? Health care provider? Frequency of check-ups? Accidents (home, work, school, driving)? (If appropriate: Storage of drugs, cleaning products, scatter rugs, etc.)
   f. In past, been easy to find ways to follow things doctors, nurses, social workers (if appropriate) suggest?
   g. Things important in family's health that I could help with?

   Examination:
   a. General appearance of family members and home.
   b. If appropriate: Storage of medicines, cribs, playpens, stove, scatter rugs, hazards, etc.

2. *Nutritional-metabolic pattern*
   History:
   a. Typical family meal pattern/food intake? (Describe.) Supplements (vitamins, types of snacks, etc.)?
   b. Typical family fluid intake? (Describe.) Supplements: type available (fruit juices, soft drinks, coffee, etc.)?
   c. Appetites?

  d. Dental problems? Dental care (frequency)?
  e. Anyone have skin problems? Healing problems?
  Examination:
  a. If opportunity available: Refrigerator contents, meal preparation, contents of meal, etc.

3. *Elimination pattern*
   History:
   a. Family use of laxatives, other aids?
   b. Problems in waste/garbage disposal?
   c. Pet animals waste disposal (indoor/outdoor)?
   d. If indicated: Problems with flies, roaches, rodents?
   Examination:
   a. If opportunity available: Examine toilet facilities, garbage disposal, pet waste disposal; indicators of risk for flies, roaches, rodents.

4. *Activity-exercise pattern*
   History:
   a. In general, does family get a lot of/little exercise? Type? Regularity?
   b. Family leisure activities? Active/passive?
   c. Problems in shopping (transportation), cooking, keeping up the house, budgeting for food, clothes, housekeeping, house costs?
   Examination:
   a. Pattern of general home maintenance, personal maintenance.

5. *Sleep-rest pattern*
   History:
   a. Generally, family members seem to be well rested and ready for school/work?
   b. Sufficient sleeping space and quiet?
   c. Family find time to relax?
   Examination:
   a. If opportunity available: Observe sleeping space and arrangements.

6. *Cognitive-perceptual pattern*
   History:
   a. Visual or hearing problems? How managed?
   b. Any big decisions family has had to make? How made?
   Examination:
   a. If indicated: Language spoken at home.
   b. Grasp of ideas and questions (abstract/concrete).
   c. Vocabulary level.

7. *Self-perception–self-concept pattern*
   History:
   a. Most of time family feels good (not so good) about themselves as a family?
   b. General mood of family? Happy? Anxious? Depressed? What helps family mood?
   Examination:
   a. General mood state: nervous (5) or relaxed (1); rate from 1 to 5.
   b. Members generally assertive (5) or passive (1); rate from 1 to 5.

8. *Role-relationship pattern*
   History:
   a. Family (or household) members? Member age and family structure (diagram).
   b. Any family problems that are difficult to handle (nuclear/extended)? Child rearing? If appropriate: Spouse ever get rough with you? The children?
   c. Relationships good (not so good) among family members? Siblings? Support each other?
   d. If appropriate: Income sufficient for needs?
   e. Feel part (or isolated) from community? Neighbors?
   Examination:
   a. Interaction among family members (if present).
   b. Observed family leadership roles.

9. *Sexuality-reproductive pattern*

History:
   a. If appropriate (sexual partner within household or situation): Sexual relations satisfying? Changes? Problems?
   b. Use of family planning? Contraceptives? Problems?
   c. If appropriate (to age of children): Feel comfortable in explaining/discussing sexual subjects?
   Examination: None

10. *Coping–stress-tolerance pattern*
   History:
   a. Any big changes within family in last few years?
   b. Family tense or relaxed most of time? When tense what helps? Anyone use medicines, drug, alcohol to decrease tension?
   c. When (if) family problems, how handled?
   d. Most of the time is this way(s) successful?
   Examination: None

11. *Value-belief pattern*
   History:
   a. Generally, family get things they want out of life?
   b. Important things for the future?
   c. Any "rules" in the family that everyone believes are important?
   d. Religion important in family? Does this help when difficulties arise?
   Examination: None

COMMUNITY ASSESSMENT*

Communities develop health patterns. In some practice settings the community is the primary client. In other cases an indi-

---

*Community assessment items are adapted from Gikow, F., & Kucharski, P. *Functional health pattern assessment of a community.* Paper presented at American Public Health Association, Proceedings of the 112th Annual Meeting, Anaheim, Cal., November 13, 1984. Gikow and Kucharski used the assessment to evaluate health-related needs of a community served by their agency.

vidual client or a family may have, or be predisposed to, certain problems that require an assessment of certain community patterns. The following are guidelines for a comprehensive community assessment, but selected patterns can also be assessed, depending on the focus of care delivery:

1. *Health-perception–health-management pattern*
   History (community representatives):
   a. In general, what is the health/wellness level of the population on a scale of 1 to 5, with 5 being high? Any major health problems?
   b. Any strong cultural patterns influencing health practices?
   c. Do people feel they have access to health services?
   d. Is there demand for any particular health services or prevention programs?
   e. Do people feel fire, police, safety programs are sufficient?
   Examination (community records):
   a. Morbidity, mortality, disability rates (by age group, if appropriate)?
   b. Accident rates (by district, if appropriate)?
   c. Currently operating health facilities (types)?
   d. Ongoing health promotion–prevention programs; utilization rates?
   e. Ratios of health professionals to population?
   f. Laws regarding drinking age?
   g. Arrest statistics for drug use/drink driving by age group?
2. *Nutritional-metabolic pattern*
   History (community representatives):
   a. In general, do most people seem well-nourished? Children? Elderly?
   b. Food supplement programs? Food stamps: Rate of use?
   c. Is cost of foods reasonable in this area relative to income?

    d. Are stores accessible for most? "Meals on Wheels" available?

    e. Water supply and quality? Testing services (if most have own wells)? (If appropriate: Water usage cost? Any drought restrictions?)

    f. Any concern that community growth will exceed good water supply?

    g. Are heating/cooling costs manageable for most? Programs?

Examination:

    a. General appearance (nutrition, teeth, clothing appropriate for climate)? Children? Adults? Elderly?

    b. Food purchases (observations at food store checkout counters)?

    c. "Junk" food (machines in schools, etc.)?

3. *Elimination pattern*

History (community representatives):

    a. Major kinds of wastes (industrial, sewage, etc.)? Disposal systems? Recycling programs? Any problems perceived by community?

    b. Pest control? Food service inspection (restaurants, street vendors, etc.)?

Examination:

    a. Communicable-disease statistics?

    b. Air pollution statistics?

4. *Activity-exercise pattern*

History (community representatives):

    a. How do people find the transportation here? To work? For recreation? To health care?

    b. Do people (senior, others) have/use community centers? Recreation facilities for children? Adults? Seniors?

    c. Is housing adequate (availability, cost)? Public housing?

Examination:

    a. Recreation/cultural programs?

    b. Aids for the disabled?

    c. Residential centers, nursing homes, rehabilitation facilities relative to population needs?

    d. External maintenance of homes, yards, apartment houses?

    e. General activity level (e.g., bustling, quiet)?

5. *Sleep-rest pattern*

History (community representatives):

    a. Generally quiet at night in most neighborhoods?

    b. Usual business hours? Are industries round-the-clock?

Examination:

    a. Activity/noise levels in business district? Residential?

6. *Cognitive-perceptual pattern*

History (community representatives):

    a. Do most groups speak English? Bilingual?

    b. Educational level of population?

    c. Schools seen as good/need improving? Adult education desired/available?

    d. Types of problems that require community decisions? Decision-making process? What is best way to get things done/changed here?

Examination:

    a. School facilities? Dropout rate?

    b. Community government structure; decision-making lines?

7. *Self-perception–self-concept pattern*

History (community representatives):

    a. Good community to live in? Going up in status, down, or about the same?

    b. Old community? Fairly new?

    c. Does any age group predominate?

    d. People's mood, in general: Enjoying life, stressed, feeling "down"?

    e. People generally have the kinds of abilities needed in this community?

f. Community/neighborhood functions? Parades?

Examination:

a. Racial, ethnic mix (if appropriate)?

b. Socioeconomic level?

c. General observations of mood?

8. *Role-relationship pattern*

History (community representatives):

a. Do people seem to get along well together here? Places where people tend to go to socialize?

b. Do people feel they are heard by the government? High/low participation in meetings?

c. Enough work/jobs for everybody? Are wages good/fair? Do people seem to like the kind of work available (happy in their jobs/job stress)?

d. Any problems with riots, violence in the neighborhoods? Family violence? Problems with child/spouse/elder abuse?

e. Does community get along with adjacent communities? Do people collaborate on any community projects?

f. Do neighbors seem to support each other?

g. Community get-togethers?

Examination:

a. Observation of interactions (generally or at specific meetings)?

b. Statistics on interpersonal violence?

c. Statistics on employment, income/poverty?

d. Divorce rate?

9. *Sexuality-reproductive pattern*

History (community representatives):

a. Average family size?

b. Do people feel there are any problems with pornography, prostitution, or other?

c. Do people want/support sex education in schools/community?

Examination:

a. Family sizes and types of households?

b. Male/female ratio?

c. Average maternal age? Maternal mortality rate? Infant mortality rate?

d. Teen pregnancy rate?

e. Abortion rate?

f. Sexual violence statistics?

g. Laws/regulations regarding information on birth control?

10. *Coping–stress-tolerance pattern*

History (community representatives):

a. Any groups that seem to be under stress?

b. Need/availability of phone help lines? Support groups (health-related, other)?

Examination:

a. Statistics on delinquency, drug abuse, alcoholism, suicide, psychiatric illness?

b. Unemployment rate by race/ethnic group/sex?

11. *Value-belief pattern*

History (community representatives):

a. Community values: What seem to be the top four things that people living here see as important in their lives? (Note health-related values, priorities.)

b. Do people tend to get involved in causes/local fund-raising campaigns? (Note if any are health-related.)

c. Are there religious groups in the community? Churches available?

d. Do people tend to tolerate/not tolerate differences or socially deviant behavior?

Examination:

a. Zoning/conservation laws?

b. Scan of community government health committee reports (goals, priorities)?

c. Health budget relative to total budget?

If a community health nurse or agency does not wish an in-depth study of a community, screening of functional patterns is possible by selecting items from the examination sections.

ASSESSMENT OF THE CRITICALLY ILL

Clients who are critically ill, such as those with *severe* respiratory, cardiac, neurological, or psychological instability, are unable to respond to a full functional health pattern assessment. At times, examination and observation are the major data collection methods used during the critical phase of an illness if the client does not have the energy, capacity, or attention span to provide a health history. Nurses caring for critically ill individuals need to use screening techniques and be sensitive to cues of high incidence diagnoses. The following may occur in homes or hospital settings:

Health perception-health management pattern
High risk for infection
High risk for injury
High risk for suffocation
Nutritional-Metabolic Pattern
High risk for nutritional deficit
High risk for pressure ulcer
Hypothermia
Ineffective thermoregulation
High risk for fluid volume deficit
High risk for aspiration
Hyperthermia
Elimination pattern
High risk for constipation/impaction
Constipation
Diarrhea
Activity-exercise pattern
High risk for activity intolerance

Activity intolerance
Ineffective airway clearance
High risk for joint contractures
Ineffective breathing pattern
Dysfunctional ventilatory weaning response (DVWR)
Total self-care deficit (Level 3-4)
Impaired bed mobility
High risk for disuse syndrome
Dysreflexia
Inability to sustain spontaneous ventilation
High risk for peripheral neurovascular dysfunction

Sleep-rest pattern

Sleep-pattern disturbance

Cognitive-perceptual pattern

Uncompensated sensory deficit (specify)
Decisional conflict
High risk for cognitive impairment
Sensory deprivation/overload
Impaired thought processes
Pain

Self-perception–self-concept pattern

Fear
Powerlessness
Self-esteem disturbance
Anxiety
Hopelessness

Role-relationship pattern

Alteration in family processes
Unresolved independence-dependence conflict
Anticipatory grieving
Dysfunctional grieving
Altered role performance
Impaired communication
Weak parent-infant attachment

Parental role conflict
Coping-Stress Tolerance Pattern
Ineffective coping
Compromised family coping
Avoidance coping
Posttrauma response
Value-Belief Pattern
Spiritual distress

USE OF DIAGNOSTIC CATEGORIES IN CLINICAL PRACTICE

Nursing diagnoses in conjunction with medical diagnoses describe the focus of most nursing care activities. Because issues of cost containment, case management, reimbursement, and quality assessment/assurance play such a large part in professional practice models, the following clinical applications of nursing diagnosis and the diagnostic categories in this manual are suggested.

1 DIAGNOSIS AND TREATMENT WITHIN NURSING PROCESS

a. Consider a diagnostic cue important until investigation of its meaning proves otherwise. A diagnostic cue is a defining characteristic (sign/symptom) of one or more diagnostic categories.

b. Use diagnostic categories as possible explanations of the meaning of cues. Consider alternative possible meanings for a cue or cue-cluster (e.g., "It's a bird; it's a plane; it's Superman").

c. Investigate the most likely possibilities first (e.g., when you see a distant speck in the sky moving toward you, think of a bird not Superman).

d. Investigate possible diagnoses by assessment of presence/absence of their critical characteristics. Critical defining characteristics are the criteria that must be present before the diagnostic label is used;

they are few in number. Research on critical characteristics is on-going.

e. Investigate the probable causes of the problem. Determine the etiological factors that, if altered, would have the greatest positive impact. Include these in the diagnostic statement; intervene on these factors first (e.g., self-care deficit, level III, related to activity intolerance).

f. Avoid premature closure; be sure sufficient cues are present to justify the diagnostic statement.

g. Syndromes do not have etiological or related factors specified. The cause is built into the diagnostic label (e.g., see posttraumatic stress, rape, translocation, disuse).

The key role of nursing diagnosis in nursing process may be seen in the diagram (pages 34-35), which depicts the components of the nursing process.

2 DOCUMENTATION

Use diagnostic category labels to describe the problem or potential problem. Use the defining characteristics to describe the cues (subjective and objective cues, if this format is employed). Etiological or related factors can document the probable cause(s) that focuses nursing care planning. (Conditions not currently labeled should be documented in descriptive terms and subjected to clinical study.) Diagnoses, diagnosis-specific interventions, and diagnosis-specific outcomes are sufficiently developed for incorporating into computerized systems.

3 COMMUNICATION

Use diagnostic category labels as concise summarizations of a cluster of cues in shift and administrative reports, discharge planning and referrals, and case conferences.

COMPONENTS OF NURSING PROCESS

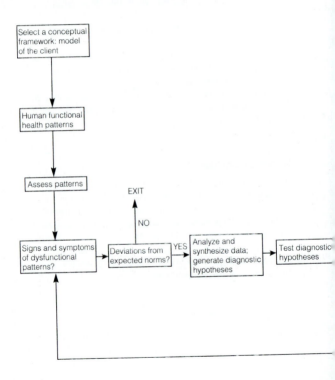

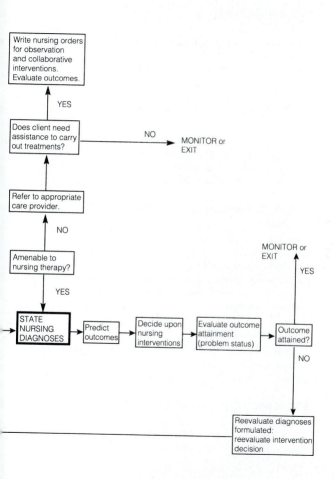

4 CONSULTATIONS

Use a set of cues and/or diagnostic category labels as concise summarizations when requesting clinical nurse specialist consultation. Diagnostic category labels are also useful when requesting consultation and specialized services to treat nursing diagnoses (e.g., nutritional, physical, occupational, recreational, art/music therapy).

5 QUALITY ASSURANCE PROGRAMS; STANDARDS OF CARE

Use diagnostic categories and their components for process and outcome audits. Assess the use of diagnoses and the accuracy of diagnostic judgments. Establish intervention and outcome standards for nursing diagnoses and criteria for their measurement.

6 COST OF NURSING CARE; REIMBURSEMENT, STAFFING

Diagnostic categories can be used as the focus of patient classification. This is necessary for costing out nursing care, reimbursement, and staffing decisions. In determining cost of services, it is necessary to obtain a refined measure of resources consumed. Cost of treatment based on nursing diagnosis, medical diagnosis, and an acuity factor is currently in the experimental stage.

7 CASE MANAGEMENT

Diagnostic category labels are used in conjunction with medical diagnoses to focus case management. Nursing diagnosis-specific outcomes are used in "outcome-focused" case management.

8 RESEARCH AND THEORY DEVELOPMENT

Diagnostic categories and their components are summarizations of concepts. They are the focus of clinical nursing research and are used in theory building within nursing science.

DOCUMENTATION: FORMAT AND EXAMPLE

Following an admission assessment, nursing diagnoses and treatment plans are documented in the client's record. Documentation is critically important for legal purposes, continuity of care, costing-out nursing services, reimbursement, and planning staffing of units.

A commonly used documentation method, the problem-oriented record, is useful for both students and expert clinicians. As the example on pages 45-49 illustrates, it includes the problem, supporting data, and the plan of care. This format for documentation provides (1) an indexing system for easy retrieval of information on a chart, (2) checkpoints for self-evaluation of diagnostic and therapeutic judgments, and (3) a master problem list (client problems listed by number) to increase coordination of treatment plans among care providers. Each diagnosis is given a number and entered on the master problem list. Following the documentation of the admission nursing history and examination, the problem number, nursing diagnosis, supporting data, and plan are recorded. Guidelines for recording are found on pages 39-41. The same problem number is used for all subsequent charting on a specific nursing diagnosis. An example of recording a nursing history and examination, diagnoses, and treatment plans may be found on pages 41-49.

Subjective or objective data related to a disease or its treatment are documented in the client's record by number (e.g., #2 Diabetes Mellitus). Relabeling of the medical problem, to chart related nursing care, is not necessary (e.g., alteration in glucose metabolism or alteration in cardiac output). In fact, relabeling in an indexing system leads to communication errors.

In some clinical settings a Kardex is used; nursing diagnoses (problem/etiology), treatments, and outcomes are listed on the Kardex. Medical diagnoses, doctors' orders, and any related nursing orders regarding observation or monitoring, drugs, treatments, and standard diagnostic and treatment protocols are also placed on the Kardex. Additional nursing orders, related to observation of disease or individualization of disease treatments, are listed on the Kardex. These nursing orders are within the collaborative domain of nursing practice and do not alter the medical treatment of disease.

With these methods of documentation, the client's record will reflect nursing judgments, actions, and evaluations relative to nursing and medical diagnoses. The Kardex will serve as a reference to all client problems that require nursing attention.

PROBLEM-ORIENTED RECORDING GUIDELINES AND CHECKPOINTS

#___ PROBLEM NUMBER AND LABEL   State clear, concise diagnostic label for the problem.

Check below that S and O contain sufficient supporting data (diagnostic criteria) for the problem.

If insufficient information available to label the problem, record the possible diagnoses being considered or major signs/symptoms; continue assessment.

S: SUBJECTIVE DATA   List pertinent diagnostic indicators from verbal reports of individual or family.

Record quotes when applicable.

Check for consistency with objective data. Attempt to resolve incongruities or inconsistencies in data before recording.

O: OBJECTIVE DATA   List pertinent diagnostic indicators from direct observation and examination of individual or family, observations of context or milieu, and observational reports of other care providers, if pertinent.

Check for measurement error, observer bias, and for consistency with subjective data. Attempt to resolve incongruities or inconsistencies in data before recording.

NOTE: S AND O DATA MUST PROVIDE SUFFICIENT DIAGNOSTIC CRITERIA TO SUPPORT PROBLEM AND ETIOLOGICAL FACTORS. SEE INDIVIDUAL DIAGNOSIS PAGES TO CHECK DEFINING CHARACTERISTICS.

A: ASSESSMENT   State etiological or related factors contributing to the problem in #_____.

Use clear, concise terms.

Check that S and O data provide diagnostic criteria for etiological factor(s).

If insufficient information available to label etiological factors, record possible factors being considered; continue assessment.

May include functional strengths pertinent to resolution of the problem and any relevant prognostic statements.

Potential problems do not have etiological factors; the risk factors recorded in S and O are the factors contributing to the high-risk state.

P: PLAN   State projected outcome(s) and interventions. PROJECTED OUTCOME(S) State concise, explicit, measurable, critical, attainable outcome(s) for the problem. State time of outcome attainment (e.g., discharge, 3 days, 4-week visit). If applicable, state a sequential set of outcomes and time frame.

Check that outcomes are specific to problem in #_____.

Check that date of outcome attainment is realistic. Consider etiological factors that may influence time for outcome attainment.

INTERVENTIONS   State intervention goal (optional). List concise nursing treatment orders. Include specific actions (time and amount, if applicable).

Check that treatment orders are consistent with cause stated in A and are specific to the individual client. If potential problem, with no etiological factor, check that treatment orders will reduce risk factors specified under S and O.

Check that treatment orders have a high possibility for attaining outcome(s).

If useful, classify plan by treatment orders (P_{RX}), diagnostic orders (P_{DX}), and teaching orders (P_{ED}).

NURSING HISTORY AND EXAMINATION

First hospital admission of 55-year-old, married, obese white male, administrator of a Spanish center. Sitting upright in bed, tense posture and expression. Five-year history of slightly elevated blood pressure. One-year PTA dizziness 12 hours and started on medication; two other episodes relieved by rest. Presents at emergency room with dizziness and numbness of left arm.

Health-Perception–Health-Management Pattern: Viewed health as good until 1 year ago when diagnosed as "having high blood pressure." States job "stressful," "but the people need me." Had headaches for last 6 months and 2 episodes of dizziness, one at work and one at home lasting about 2 hours. Rested and symptoms went away. Delayed seeking care because was "too busy." Thought it was "overwork," not blood pressure. Discontinued blood pressure medication and M.D. visits about 6 months ago: "When blood pressure came down and I felt better"; states medicine caused impotence. To emergency room today because of left arm numbness and fear of stroke. Mother died of "stroke" 15 months ago. Concerned that he hasn't been taking care of himself and "I need to learn about what to do." Wants to know "everything."

Asked if O.K. to do some job-related paper work if someone brought it in. Takes no medicine currently, except Alka-Seltzer and a laxative; doesn't smoke; social drinking.

Nutritional-Metabolic Pattern: Sample diet related: MDR intake of protein, excess carbohydrate and fat; minimal high roughage foods (fruits and vegetables), approximately 3 c coffee/day, fluid intake low, no history of lesions at mouth corners or mucous membranes; has gained weight gradually last 15 years. Some indigestion and heartburn after lunch attributed to days with multiple problems; takes Alka-Seltzer; dieting unsuccessful; problem is "probably stress of job; I get home and eat big supper and snacks in evening"; no food dislikes. Takes lunch (sandwich and cake) to work and eats at desk; restaurants in area not good.

Elimination Pattern: Daily bowel movement pattern with 2-3 episodes of constipation/month lasting 2 days, hard stools, straining, and laxatives used. Attributes this pattern to his diet; knows he should eat better. Reports no problems voiding or in control of elimination.

Activity-Exercise Pattern: Spectator sports, uses car, minimal walking due to time schedule, sedentary job, considers self too old for exercise. Increasing fatigue last few weeks, less energy 2 months before admission; no self-care deficit. Recreation consists of reading novels, watching T.V., dinner with other couples. Lives in first-floor apartment in city and drives ¾ mile to work.

Sleep-Rest Pattern: Average 4-6 hours sleep/night, quiet atmosphere, own room with wife, double bed, uses bed board. Pre-sleep activities include watching T.V. or completing paper work from job; difficulty with sleep onset 1 month; awakens in morning many times thinking about job-related problems.

Cognitive-Perceptual Pattern: Sight corrected with glasses, changed 1 year ago; no change in hearing, taste, smell. No perceived change in memory; "I couldn't take it if I started losing my mind, like with a stroke." Learning ability: sees self as slower than in college, alert manner, grasps questions easily. Takes no sedatives, tranquilizers, other drugs. No headache at present.

Self-Perception–Self-Concept Pattern: Sees self as needing to do things well (job, father, husband); "sometimes don't think I'm doing well with my family having them live in this area, but in my job you have to be near when people need help." "It will be just great if I get sick and they have to take care of me, instead of me taking care of them."

Role-Relationship Pattern: Describes family as happy and understanding of his job commitments, wife former social worker; "kids good"; "but I know we'll have trouble as Joe (10 years old) gets older"; "maybe I should move out of [lower socioeco area in city cited]." 10-year-old assaulted 4 months ago; 14-year-old boy interested in sports and "keeps out of trouble, so far." Family usually "sits down together" to handle problems. Social relationships confined to "a few other couples," finds this sufficient. Job demanding 9-10 hours/day "always trying to get money to keep the center solvent" (assistant taking over while in hospital); enjoys job and helping people; coworkers are "good to work with." Wife states they are close; worried about husband's health; states he is more concerned with other people than himself; she admires him for this. Wife able to handle home responsibilities during hospitalization. States she and children had physical exam recently; no health problems; no elevation in blood pressure.

Sexuality-Reproductive Pattern: Two children; states impotent when on BP medication. When "BP went down" stopped meds;

potency returned. No problems perceived in sexual relationship.
Coping–Stress-Tolerance Pattern: Feels tense at work; has tried
relaxation exercises with some alleviation; doesn't always have
time. States the best way to deal with problems is to "attack
them." Afraid of having a stroke and being dependent; "this
thing today has really scared me." "I have too many things to
think about at work and at home and now this blood pressure
thing." Life changes: Father died 3 years ago; mother died of
stroke 15 months ago. Took job at Spanish center 2 years ago to
be near mother who "was getting old." Pleased he did this and
feels good about it.
Value-Belief Pattern: "Life has been good to me"; feels deeply
about "injustices in society" and wants to do something about
them. States family is important to him. Religion (Catholic) important to him; would like to be active in church affairs.

Examination
Blood pressure _____205/118_____ Temperature _____99.8_____
Pulse rate ___regular and strong___ Respirations _____18_____
Nutritional-Metabolic Pattern
Skin No area of redness over bony prominences; no lesions.
Dryness, callouses on feet, and discomfort.
Oral mucous membranes Moist, no lesions.
Actual wt _____230_____ Reported wt _____220_____ Ht ___5'11"___
Activity-Exercise Pattern
Activity-Exercise Pattern
Gait ___Steady___ Posture ___Well balanced___
Muscle tone, strength-coordination Hand grip firm left and
right; lifts legs; can pick up pencil; tenseness in neck and shoul-
der muscles.
Range of motion (joints) Some tightness in bending forward
Prostheses-assistive devices _____None_____
Absence of body part ___No___

Demonstrated ability for:

Feeding ____0____ Grooming ____0____

Bathing ____0____ General mobility ____0____

Toileting ____0____ Dressing ____0____

(0 = full self-care)

Cognitive-Perceptual Pattern

Perceptual: Hears whisper ____Yes____ Reads newsprint __with__
glasses

Language: __English; grasps ideas, abstract and concrete;__
__speech clear; attention span good__

Self-Perception–Self-Concept Pattern

General appearance __Well groomed, good hygiene__

Nervous/relaxed __2 (scale of 1-5) Tense; some relaxation__
__during history taking__

Eye contact ____Yes____ Attention span ____Good____

Assertive/Passive __3 (scale of 1-5)__

Role-Relationship Pattern

Interactions: __Communications with wife supportive; both__
__somewhat tense, children not present.__

PROBLEM LIST

1. Exogenous Obesity

    S: Reports diet with excess carbohydrate and fat; big sup-
    per, snacks in evening, sandwich and cake at lunch,
    eats at desk. Reports gradual weight gain last 15 years;
    considers self too old for exercise; sedentary job; spec-
    tator sports, drives ¾ mile to work. Reports 220 lbs.

    O: 5'11", 230 lbs. Dryness, callouses on feet with dis-
    comfort when walking. Current diet order: 1200 calo-
    ries.

    A: Caloric Intake-Energy Expenditure Imbalance. Reports
    dieting unsuccessful in past; discomfort when walking
    may reduce exercise.

Discharge Outcome: (1) Writes one week's 1200 calorie diet using calorie guide; (2) States how meal plan can be carried out within daily routine; (3) States plan for increasing exercise and amount of weight loss to be achieved per month.

P: Discuss why dieting previously unsuccessful. Assess motivation, readiness, and current plans for weight loss; develop educational plan to achieve outcomes. Suggest podiatrist.

2. Intermittent Constipation Pattern

S: Daily bowel movement with 2-3 episodes of constipation per month; constipation lasts 2 days, hard stools, straining, laxatives used; attributes this to minimal high roughage foods, low fluid intake; minimal walking, exercise; no constipation reported at present.

A: Dietary-Exercise Pattern

Discharge Outcome: (1) Daily bowel movement without straining. (2) States a plan for increasing fluid intake and high fiber foods in diet.

P: Check qd bowel pattern in hospital. Provide supplementary fluids between meals. Integrate teaching of fluid and high fiber food requirements into weight loss dietary teaching (see 1).

3. Fear (dependency)

S: "Couldn't take it if it started losing my mind, like with a stroke"; "just great if I get sick and they have to take care of me, instead of me care for them," states fear of stroke and becoming dependent—"this today has scared me"; mother died of stroke 15 months ago. States best way to deal with problems is to "attack them."

O: Neck and shoulder muscles tense

A: Perceived risk of stroke

Outcome, Day 2: (1) Neck and shoulder muscles relaxed, (2) Identifies ways to reduce future risk of dependency (stroke).

P: Orient to environment and explain procedures (cognitive and sensory orientation).

Back massage for relaxation q4h times 2 days. Allow to verbalize fears of dependency and channel thinking toward "attacking" risk factors; integrate discussion with dietary planning and conflict resolution.

4. Value Conflict

S: Feels deeply about injustices in society; wants to do something about them; head of Spanish Center in inner city; enjoys job and helping people; coworkers good; job demanding, 9–10 hrs./day; always trying to get money to keep solvent; "job stressful, but people need me"; feels tense at work—tried relaxation; doesn't always have time to relax; 4-6 hrs. sleep/night, sleep onset difficulty 1 month, presleep activities include job-related paper work; awakens thinking about job-related problems.

Wife states he's more concerned with others than himself—admires him for this; "kids good, but know we'll have trouble as Joe gets older"; "maybe I should move"; 10-year old assaulted 4 months ago; sees self as needing to do things well (job, father, husband); sometimes thinks "not doing well with family—having them live in this area; but in my job you have to be near when people need help." "I have too many things to think about at work, at home, and now this blood pressure thing."

O: BP 205/118; 5-yr. history of essential hypertension.

A: Perceived responsibilities (job and family, possibly self)

Discharge Outcome: States plan for periodically assessing
   commitments/priorities in life.
P: Assess time constraints relative to valued activities
   (job, family, health management responsibilities).
   Help determine high-priority responsibilities (clarify
   values).
      Discuss possibility that time allocation to valued
      areas may resolve conflicts.
      Discuss value of health management so can continue
      to help others and realize goals.
      Consider nursing referral.

5. High-Risk Health Management Deficit*
   S: Delayed seeking care because "too busy"; attributed
      headaches and dizziness to overwork; stopped meds
      and follow-up care when "BP went down"; states im-
      potent on BP meds.
   O: BP 205/118; 5'11", 230 lbs.
   A: May be motivated to improve health management at
      this time; states wants to learn what to do.
   Discharge Outcome: States how daily routine will be
      adapted to implement health management plans (medi-
      cation regimen, diet–exercise, bowel, and value-con-
      flict management)
   P: Assess motivation and readiness to improve health
      management; develop plan for learning the manage-
      ment of hypertension, diet, exercise, elimination, and
      value conflict (the general plan of hypertensive and
      transient-ischemic attack management can be reviewed
      until specific drugs, etc., are prescribed for discharge)
6. Hypertension with Evidence of Transient Ischemic Attack
   (medical diagnosis made and recorded by physician)

*It may be possible to cluster all other problems under Health Management Def-
icit/Perceived Responsibilities and Priorities. The care objective would be to
help the client balance job, family, and health management responsibilities.

P: Allopurinal 300 mgm bid; 1200 calorie diet with no
added salt BP q4h, notify M.D. if diastolic greater
than 120, severe headache, dizziness (medical orders)
Observe for weakness in muscles of face or extremities
and notify M.D. (nursing order).

LEGAL CONSIDERATIONS IN NURSING DIAGNOSIS

The legal implications of using the diagnostic categories contained in
this manual deserve attention. Nurses have a legal duty (as well as a
moral duty) to prevent harm to clients. Harm resulting from the nurse's
action or inaction can be the basis of a malpractice claim. Diagnoses and
diagnostic judgments may enter the picture when the question is raised:
Why did the harm occur?

Making a nursing diagnosis can help prevent harm to patients. Diagnostic judgments bring to conscious awareness the presence of a problem/
risk factor that requires nursing intervention. Careful assessment, thoughtful diagnosis, wise treatment decisions, care implemented safely, and ac-
curate documentation reduce the possibility of harm to patients and legal
judgments of negligence against nurses.

Harm can be caused by negligent conduct on the part of a nurse in
care delivery or in delegation and supervision of others' care delivery. A
legal judgment of malpractice can result and may carry a severe financial
settlement against a nurse, suspension or loss of a nurse's license to practice, or both. (This is in addition to the emotional trauma.) Negligence in
diagnosis and treatment can be established if the nurse had an element of
duty to the patient and a breach of duty occurred. Legally the element of
duty is specified in state nurse practice acts and is further supported by
professional standards of practice and a social policy statement (American
Nurses' Association, 1974; 1980). Two other conditions for negligence
that have to be established are harm or injury and cause and effect. It has
to be demonstrated that actual injury and loss occurred (physical, psychological, or both), including economic loss. Also, a cause and effect rela-

tionship between the nurse's conduct and an alleged injury has to be established.

Development of clinical judgment skills and knowledge of diagnostic categories will help to avoid errors of omission (failing to intervene when a nursing diagnosis is present) and errors of commission (taking harmful nursing actions when a condition is not present because of overdiagnosing or incorrect diagnosis). Responsibility and accountability are clear in nursing's social policy statement to consumers (American Nurses' Association, 1980). Nursing is described as the "diagnosis and treatment of human responses to actual or potential health problems" (dysfunctional health patterns). Professional nurses assume legal accountability for accuracy in diagnosis and for interventions and outcomes for nursing diagnoses. Further discussion of this topic can be found in (Gordon, 1987).

American Nurses' Association: *Nursing: A social policy statement,* Kansas City, Mo, 1980, The Association.
Gordon M: *Nursing diagnosis: Process and application,* ed. 2, St Louis, 1987, Mosby—Year Book.

DIAGNOSTIC CATEGORIES

HEALTH-PERCEPTION–
HEALTH-MANAGEMENT
PATTERN

NOTES

Altered Health Maintenance

DEFINITION
☐ Inability to identify, manage, or seek help to maintain health

DEFINING CHARACTERISTICS
☐ Demonstrated lack of knowledge regarding basic health practices
☐ Demonstrated lack of adaptive behaviors to internal or external changes
☐ Reported or observed inability to take responsibility for meeting basic health practices in any, or all, functional pattern areas
☐ Reported or observed lack of equipment, finances, or other resources for health maintenance
☐ Reported or observed impairment of personal support system
☐ History of lack of health seeking behavior
☐ Expression of interest in improving health behaviors

ETIOLOGICAL OR RELATED FACTORS
☐ Alteration or lack of communication skills (written, verbal, gestural)
☐ Inability to make deliberative and thoughtful judgments
☐ Perceptual-cognitive impairment
☐ Complete or partial lack of gross/fine motor skills
☐ Ineffective coping (individual or family)
☐ Disabling spiritual distress
☐ Lack of material resources
☐ Unachieved developmental tasks
☐ Dysfunctional grieving

NOTES

Ineffective Management of Therapeutic Regimen

DEFINITION
- Pattern of regulating/integrating into daily living a program for treating illness and sequelae of illness that is not meeting specific health goals

DEFINING CHARACTERISTICS
- Choices of daily living ineffective for meeting goals of a treatment or prevention program (specify)
- Acceleration (expected or unexpected) of illness symptoms
- Expresses desire to manage the treatment of illness/prevention of sequelae
- Verbalizes difficulty with regulation/integration of one or more prescribed regimens for treatment of illness/illness effects/prevention of complications
- States that did not take action to include treatment regimens in daily routines
- States did not take action to reduce risk factors for progression of illness and sequelae

ETIOLOGICAL OR RELATED FACTORS
- Low perceived seriousness
- Perceived low susceptibility
- Perceived barriers (specify)
- Perceived cost exceeds benefits
- Mistrust (specify [e.g., of regimen/health care personnel])
- Powerlessness
- Complexity of therapeutic regimen

(Continued)

NOTES

Ineffective Management of Therapeutic Regimen *Continued*

- ☐ Decisional conflict (specify)
- ☐ Economic difficulties
- ☐ Excessive demands made on individual/family
- ☐ Family conflict
- ☐ Family patterns of health care (specify)
- ☐ Inadequate cues to action (number/types)
- ☐ Knowledge deficit (Specify)
- ☐ Social support deficits
- ☐ Complexity of health care system

*See also Noncompliance, Health Management Deficit, Altered Health Maintenance.

NOTES

Total Health Management Deficit

DEFINITION

☐ Inability to manage own disease treatment or health promotion activities. (Refers to total health management deficit, including disease treatment and observations.) For partial deficits use Health Management Deficit (Specify).

DEFINING CHARACTERISTICS

☐ Knowledge, comprehension, and/or motor skills required for continuing treatment of disease exceed actual or potential competencies

☐ Knowledge, comprehension, and/or motor skills required for disease prevention and health promotion exceed actual or potential competencies

ETIOLOGICAL OR RELATED FACTORS

☐ Activity intolerance (level IV)
☐ Uncompensated perceptual or cognitive impairment
☐ Uncompensated impaired coordination
☐ Impaired mobility (level II-IV)
☐ Uncompensated short-term memory deficit
☐ Impaired reality testing
☐ Severe depression
☐ Parental care priorities
☐ Priority setting

NOTES

Health Management Deficit (Specify)

DEFINITION
- Inability to manage aspects of own disease treatment or health promotion activities. (Specify area of deficit, e.g., drug or treatment regime, dietary prescription, observation and reporting of symptoms, follow-up care of disease, health promotion activities.)

DEFINING CHARACTERISTICS
- Knowledge, comprehension, and/or motor skills required for aspects of continuing treatment of disease exceed actual or potential competencies.
- Knowledge, comprehension, and/or motor skills required for specific health promotion and disease prevention activities exceed actual or potential competencies.

ETIOLOGICAL OR RELATED FACTORS
- Activity intolerance (Level IV)
- Uncompensated perceptual or cognitive impairment
- Uncompensated impaired coordination
- Impaired mobility (Level II-IV)
- Uncompensated short-term memory deficit
- Uncompensated visual or hearing loss
- Impaired reality testing
- Severe depression

NOTES

Noncompliance (Specify)

DEFINITION

☐ Nonadherence to a therapeutic recommendation following informed decision and expressed intention to attain therapeutic goals

DEFINING CHARACTERISTICS

☐ *Direct observation of noncompliance
☐ *Statements by client or significant others describing noncompliance
☐ Objective tests revealing noncompliance (physiological measures, detection of markers)
☐ Evidence of development of complications
☐ Evidence of exacerbation of symptoms
☐ Failure to keep appointments
☐ Failure to progress (resolve problem)

ETIOLOGICAL OR RELATED FACTORS

☐ Value conflict
☐ Cultural conflict
☐ Spiritual conflict
☐ Knowledge or skill deficit
☐ Perceived therapeutic ineffectiveness
☐ Perceived nonsusceptibility or invulnerability
☐ Denial of illness
☐ Family pattern disruption

NOTES

High Risk for Noncompliance (Specify)

DEFINITION
☐ Presence of risk factors for nonadherence to the therapeutic recommendations following expressed intention to adhere or attain therapeutic goals

DEFINING CHARACTERISTICS (RISK FACTORS)
☐ History of noncompliance with aspects of therapeutic regime
☐ Lack of support systems (supportive others)
☐ Denial of illness
☐ Perceived ineffectiveness of recommended practices
☐ Perceived lack of seriousness of problem or risk factors
☐ Perceived lack of susceptibility
☐ Insufficient knowledge or skills (therapeutic recommendations)
☐ Absence of a plan for integrating therapeutic recommendations into daily routines

NOTES

Potential Noncompliance (Specify)

DEFINITION

- Presence of risk factors for nonadherence to therapeutic recommendations following expressed intention to adhere or attain therapeutic goals

DEFINING CHARACTERISTICS (RISK FACTORS)

- History of noncompliance with aspects of therapeutic regime
- Lack of support systems (supportive others)
- Denial of illness
- Perceived ineffectiveness of recommended practices
- Perceived lack of seriousness of problem or risk factors
- Perceived lack of susceptibility
- Insufficient knowledge or skills (therapeutic recommendations)
- Absence of a plan for integrating therapeutic recommendations into daily routines

NOTES

High Risk for Infection

DEFINITION

☐ The state in which an individual is at increased risk for invasion by pathogenic organisms

DEFINING CHARACTERISTICS (RISK FACTORS)

☐ Inadequate primary defenses (broken skin, traumatized tissues, decrease in ciliary action, stasis of body fluids, change in pH of secretions, altered peristalsis)
☐ Inadequate secondary defenses (e.g., decreased hemoglobin, leukopenia, suppressed inflammatory response)
☐ Immunosuppression
☐ Inadequate acquired immunity
☐ Insufficient knowledge to avoid exposure to pathogens
☐ Tissue destruction and increased environmental exposure
☐ Chronic disease
☐ Invasive procedures
☐ Malnutrition
☐ Pharmaceutical agents and trauma
☐ Rupture of amniotic membranes

NOTES

High Risk for Injury (Trauma)

DEFINITION
☐ Presence of risk factors for bodily injury

DEFINING CHARACTERISTICS (RISK FACTORS)
☐ Disorientation
☐ Impaired judgment (disease, drugs, reality testing, risk-taking behavior)
☐ Muscle weakness, paralysis, incoordination; balancing difficulties; mobility impairment
☐ Sensory-perceptual deterioration (temperature, touch, position-sense, vision, hearing)
☐ History of previous trauma, accidental injury (falling, car accidents)
☐ Insufficient finances to purchase safety equipment or effect repairs
☐ Lack of safety precautions, safety education
☐ Excess alcohol-ingestion pattern
☐ Altered blood-clotting factors (bleeding tendency)
☐ Slippery, littered, or obstructed floors, stairs, walkways (wet, highly waxed, snow, ice)
☐ Unanchored rugs, unsturdy or absent stair rails; unsteady ladders or chairs
☐ Bathtub without hand grips or anti-slip equipment
☐ Entering unlighted rooms
☐ Unanchored electric wires
☐ High beds
☐ Children playing without gates at top of stairs
☐ Unsafe window protection in homes with young children
☐ Sliding on coarse bed linen and struggling within bed restraints
(Continued)

NOTES

High Risk for Injury *Continued*

- ☐ Smoking in bed or near oxygen
- ☐ Inappropriate call-for-aid mechanisms for bed-resting client
- ☐ Pot handles facing toward front of stove
- ☐ Bathing in very hot water; unsupervised bathing of young children
- ☐ Potential igniting gas leaks; delayed lighting of gas burner or oven; grease waste collected on stoves
- ☐ Use of thin or worn potholders or mitts
- ☐ Experimenting with chemicals or gasoline; contact with acid or alkali
- ☐ Play or work near vehicle pathways (driveways, laneways, railroad tracks)
- ☐ Children playing with matches, candles, cigarettes, fire-works, gunpowder, sharp-edged toys
- ☐ Inadequately stored combustible or corrosive materials (matches, oily rags, lye)
- ☐ Children riding in front seat of automobile; unrestrained babies riding in car
- ☐ Highly flammable children's toys or clothing
- ☐ Overloaded fuse boxes or electrical outlets; faulty electrical plugs; frayed wires; defective appliances
- ☐ Exposure to dangerous machinery, contact with rapidly moving machinery, industrial belts, pulleys
- ☐ Overexposure to sun, sun lamps
- ☐ Use of cracked dishware or glasses; knives stored uncovered
- ☐ Guns or ammunition stored unlocked
- ☐ Large icicles hanging from roof
- ☐ High-crime neighborhood *(Continued)*

NOTES

High Risk for Injury   *Continued*

- ☐ Unsafe roads or road-crossing conditions
- ☐ Driving mechanically unsafe vehicles; driving after partaking of alcoholic beverages, drugs
- ☐ Driving at excessive speeds or without necessary visual aids
- ☐ Non-use or misuse of seat restraints, headgear for cyclists and passengers

NOTES

High Risk for Poisoning

DEFINITION

☐ Presence of risk factors for accidental exposure to, or ingestion of, drugs or dangerous products in doses sufficient to cause poisoning

DEFINING CHARACTERISTICS (RISK FACTORS)

☐ Reduced vision
☐ Occupational setting without adequate safeguards
☐ Lack of safety or drug education
☐ Cognitive impairment or emotional difficulties
☐ Insufficient finances
☐ Large supplies of drugs in the house
☐ Medicines stored in unlocked cabinets accessible to children or confused persons
☐ Dangerous products placed or stored within reach of children or confused persons
☐ Availability of illicit drug potentially contaminated by poisonous additives
☐ Flaking, peeling paint or plaster in presence of young children
☐ Chemical contamination of food or water
☐ Unprotected contact with heavy metals or chemicals
☐ Paint, lacquer, etc., in poorly ventilated areas or without effective protection
☐ Presence of poisonous vegetation
☐ Presence of atmospheric pollutants

NOTES

High Risk for Suffocation

DEFINITION

☐ Presence of risk factors for accidental interruption in air available for inhalation

DEFINING CHARACTERISTICS (RISK FACTORS)

☐ Reduced olfactory sensation
☐ Cognitive impairment or emotional difficulties
☐ Mobility impairment (bed mobility or ambulation)
☐ Lack of safety education or safety precaution
☐ Vehicle warming in a closed garage
☐ Pillow placed in an infant's crib
☐ Propped bottle placed in an infant's crib
☐ Pacifier hung around an infant's head
☐ Children playing in plastic bags, inserting small objects into their mouths or noses
☐ Discarded or unused refrigerators; freezers without removed doors
☐ Children left unattended in bathtubs, pools
☐ Household gas leaks
☐ Use of fuel-burning heaters not vented to the outside
☐ Eating large mouthfuls of food

NOTES

Altered Protection

DEFINITION
- Decreased ability to guard self from internal or external threats such as illness or injury

DEFINING CHARACTERISTICS (RISK FACTORS)
- Deficient immunity
- Impaired healing
- Altered clotting
- Maladaptive stress response
- Neurosensory alterations
- Chilling, perspiring
- Dyspnea, cough
- Itching
- Restlessness
- Insomnia, fatigue, anorexia, weakness
- Immobility
- Disorientation
- Pressure sores

ETIOLOGICAL OR RELATED FACTORS
- Inadequate nutrition
- Alcohol abuse
- Abnormal blood profiles (leukopenia, thrombocytopenia, anemia, coagulation)
- Drug therapies (antineoplastic, corticosteroid, immune, anticoagulant, thrombolytic)
- Treatments (surgery, radiation, cancer, immune disorders)

NOTES

NUTRITIONAL-METABOLIC PATTERN

NOTES

Altered Nutrition: High Risk for More than Body Requirements *or High Risk for Obesity*

DEFINITION

☐ Presence of risk factors for excess caloric intake relative to metabolic need

DEFINING CHARACTERISTICS (RISK FACTORS)

☐ *Reported or observed obesity in one or both parents; hereditary predisposition
☐ *Rapid transition across growth percentiles in infants or children
☐ Excessive intake relative to energy expenditure during late gestational life, early infancy, and adolescence
☐ Dysfunctional eating patterns:
  a. Pairing food with other activities
  b. Concentrating food intake at end of day
  c. Eating in response to external cues (time of day, social situation)
  d. Eating in response to internal cues (anxiety, depression)
☐ Sedentary activity level
☐ Dysfunctional psychological conditioning in response to food (use of food as reward or comfort measure)
☐ Frequent closely spaced pregnancies; reported or observed higher baseline right at beginning of each pregnancy
☐ Low financial resources (selection of lower cost high-caloric foods)

NOTES

Altered Nutrition: More than Body Requirements *or Exogenous Obesity*

DEFINITION
☐ Excess caloric intake relative to metabolic need

DEFINING CHARACTERISTICS
☐ *Weight 20% over ideal for height and frame
☐ *Triceps skin fold greater than 15 mm in men and 25 mm in women
☐ Weight 10% over ideal for height and frame
☐ Sedentary activity level

ETIOLOGICAL OR RELATED FACTORS
☐ Food intake-energy expenditure imbalance
☐ Dysfunctional eating patterns (reported or observed)
   a. Pairing food with other activities
   b. Concentrating food intake at end of day
   c. Eating in response to external cues (time of day, social situation)
   d. Eating in response to internal cues other than hunger (anxiety, depression)

NOTES

Altered Nutrition: Less than Body Requirements *or Nutritional Deficit (Specify)*

DEFINITION
- Insufficient intake of nutrients to meet metabolic needs

DEFINING CHARACTERISTICS
- Twenty percent or more under ideal body weight
- Reported or observed inadequate food intake relative to minimum daily requirements
- Weight loss (with or without adequate intake)
- Capillary fragility
- Pale conjunctiva and mucous membranes
- Fatigue
- Excessive hair loss; poor muscle tone
- Hyperactive bowel sounds; abdominal cramping, pain
- Diarrhea and/or steatorrhea

ETIOLOGICAL OR RELATED FACTORS
- Buccal cavity discomfort/pain
- Pain with mastication (dental caries)
- Altered taste sensation
- Inability to prepare/procure food
- Diarrhea, steatorrhea
- Knowledge deficit (daily requirements)
- Financial limitations
- Edentulous
- Social isolation

(Continued)

NOTES

Altered Nutrition: Less than Body Requirements *or Nutritional Deficit* Continued

- ☐ Anorexia, setophobia, early satiety
- ☐ Chemical dependency
- ☐ Emotional stress
- ☐ Food faddism, dieting practices
- ☐ Muscle weakness (mastication, swallowing)

NOTES

Ineffective Breastfeeding

DEFINITION
☐ Dissatisfaction or difficulty with the breastfeeding process experienced by mother or infant/child

DEFINING CHARACTERISTICS
☐ Actual/perceived inadequate milk supply
☐ Infant inability to attach to maternal breast correctly
☐ No observable signs of oxytocin release
☐ Observable signs of inadequate infant intake
☐ Nonsustained/insufficient opportunity for suckling at the breast
☐ Insufficient emptying of each breast per feeding
☐ Persistence of sore nipples beyond the first week of breastfeeding
☐ Infant exhibiting fussiness and crying within first hour after breastfeeding; unresponsive to comfort measures
☐ Infant arching and crying at the breast; resisting latching on
☐ Previous history of breastfeeding failure

ETIOLOGICAL OR RELATED FACTORS
☐ Knowledge deficit (breastfeeding)
☐ Interrupted breastfeeding
☐ Maternal anxiety; maternal ambivalence
☐ Prematurity or infant anomaly
☐ Maternal breast anomaly; previous breast surgery
☐ Infant supplemental feedings with artificial nipple
☐ Poor infant sucking reflex
☐ Nonsupportive partner/family

NOTES

Effective Breastfeeding*

DEFINITION

☐ Mother-infant dyad/family exhibits adequate proficiency and satisfaction with breastfeeding process.

DEFINING CHARACTERISTICS

☐ *Mother able to position infant at breast to promote a successful latch-on response
☐ *Infant is content after feeding
☐ *Regular and sustained suckling/swallowing at the breast
☐ *Appropriate infant weight patterns for age
☐ *Effective mother/infant communication patterns (infant cues; maternal interpretation and response)
☐ Signs/symptoms of oxytocin release (let down or milk ejection reflex)
☐ Adequate infant elimination patterns for age
☐ Eagerness of infant to nurse
☐ Maternal verbalization of satisfaction with the breastfeeding process

ETIOLOGICAL OR RELATED FACTORS

☐ Basic breastfeeding knowledge
☐ Normal breast structure
☐ Normal infant oral structure
☐ Infant gestational age greater than 34 weeks
☐ Support sources
☐ Maternal confidence

*This diagnostic category does not represent a problem or high risk. As with other healthy states or processes, periodic assessment is advisable.

NOTES

Interrupted Breastfeeding

DEFINITION
☐ Break in continuity of breastfeeding process as a result of inability or inadvisability to put baby to breast for feeding

DEFINING CHARACTERISTICS
☐ *Infant does not receive nourishment at the breast for some or all of the feedings
☐ Maternal desire to maintain lactation and provide (or eventually provide) her breastmilk for infant's nutritional needs
☐ Lack of knowledge regarding expression and storage of breastmilk

ETIOLOGICAL OR RELATED FACTORS
☐ Mother-infant separation
☐ Maternal or infant illness
☐ Maternal employment
☐ Contraindications to breastfeeding (e.g., drugs, true breastmilk jaundice)
☐ Need to abruptly wean infant
☐ Prematurity

NOTES

Ineffective Infant Feeding Pattern

DEFINITION
- ☐ Infant demonstrates an impaired ability to suck or coordinate the suck-swallow response

DEFINING CHARACTERISTICS
- ☐ *Inability to initiate or sustain an effective suck
- ☐ *Inability to coordinate sucking, swallowing, or breathing

ETIOLOGICAL OR RELATED FACTORS
- ☐ Prematurity
- ☐ Neurological impairment/delay (specify)
- ☐ Oral hypersensitivity
- ☐ Prolonged NPO
- ☐ Anatomic abnormality (specify)

NOTES

High Risk for Aspiration

DEFINITION
☐ Presence of risk factors for entry of gastrointestinal secretions, oropharyngeal secretions, solids, or fluids into tracheobronchial passage

DEFINING CHARACTERISTICS (RISK FACTORS)
☐ Episodes of choking on secretions, food, or fluids
☐ Reduced level of consciousness
☐ Depressed cough and gag reflexes
☐ Presence of tracheostomy, endotracheal, or gastrointestinal tube
☐ Tube feedings
☐ Situations hindering elevation of upper body
☐ Facial/oral/neck surgery or trauma
☐ Wired jaws
☐ Incomplete lower esophageal sphincter
☐ Increased intragastric pressure
☐ Increased gastric residual
☐ Decreased gastrointestinal motility
☐ Delayed gastric emptying
☐ Medication administration

NOTES

Impaired Swallowing *or*
Uncompensated Swallowing Impairment

DEFINITION

☐ The state in which an individual has decreased ability to voluntarily pass fluids and/or solids from the mouth to the stomach

DEFINING CHARACTERISTICS

☐ *Observed evidence of difficulty in swallowing:
  Stasis of food in oral cavity (cheek pocket)
  Coughing/choking when swallowing
☐ Evidence of aspiration

ETIOLOGICAL OR RELATED FACTORS

☐ Neuromuscular impairment:
  Decreased or absent gag reflex
  Decreased strength or excursion of muscles involved in mastication
  Perceptual impairment
  Facial paralysis
☐ Mechanical obstruction:
  Edema
  Tracheostomy tube
  Tumor
☐ Fatigue
☐ Limited awareness
☐ Reddened, irritated oropharyngeal cavity

NOTES

Altered Oral Mucous Membrane

DEFINITION
☐ Change in secretions, membranes, or structures of the oral cavity producing pain or discomfort

DEFINING CHARACTERISTICS
☐ Verbalization or signs of pain or discomfort in oral mucous membranes
☐ Decrease in or lack of saliva
☐ Coated tongue; xerostomia (dry mouth)
☐ Halitosis
☐ Edema of membranes; hyperemia
☐ Oral lesions: ulcers, desquamation, vesicles, hemorrhagic gingivitis, leukoplakia
☐ Stomatitis
☐ Oral plaque
☐ Carious teeth

ETIOLOGICAL OR RELATED FACTORS
☐ Ineffective oral hygiene
☐ Malnutrition, dehydration
☐ Intake restrictions (NPO greater than 24 hours)
☐ Mouth breathing
☐ Decreased (absent) salivation
☐ Chemical irritants (acidic foods, drugs, noxious agents, alcohol)
☐ Mechanical irritants (ill-fitting dentures, braces, endotracheal or nasogastric tubes; surgery to oral cavity)
☐ Trauma
☐ Oral cavity radiation (head and neck)
☐ Infections

NOTES

High Risk for Fluid Volume Deficit

DEFINITION
☐ Presence of risk factors for decrease in body fluid (vascular, cellular, or intracellular dehydration)

DEFINING CHARACTERISTICS (RISK FACTORS)
☐ Extremes of age
☐ Extremes of weight
☐ Excessive loss of fluid through normal routes (e.g., diarrhea)
☐ Loss of fluid through abnormal routes (e.g., indwelling tubes)
☐ Deviations affecting access to fluids, intake of fluids, or absorption of fluids (e.g., physical immobility, unconsciousness)
☐ Factors influencing fluid requirements (e.g., hypermetabolic states; hyperthermia; dry, hot environment)
☐ Knowledge deficit related to fluid volume needs
☐ Medications (e.g., diuretics)
☐ Increased fluid output
☐ Urinary frequency
☐ Thirst

NOTES

Fluid Volume Deficit

DEFINITION

The state in which an individual experiences vascular, cellular, or intracellular dehydration.

DEFINING CHARACTERISTICS

- ☐ Change in urine output
- ☐ Change in urine concentration
- ☐ Thirst
- ☐ Sudden weight loss or gain
- ☐ Decreased venous filling
- ☐ Hemoconcentration; change in serum sodium
- ☐ Hypotension; decreased pulse volume/pressure
- ☐ Increased pulse rate
- ☐ Decreased skin turgor
- ☐ Dry skin; dry mucous membranes
- ☐ Change in mental state
- ☐ Increased body temperature
- ☐ Weakness

ETIOLOGICAL OR RELATED FACTORS

- ☐ Active fluid volume loss
- ☐ Failure of regulatory mechanisms

NOTES

Fluid Volume Excess[1]

DEFINITION
☐ Increased local or total body fluid volume

DEFINING CHARACTERISTICS
☐ Edema, effusion, anasarca
☐ Sudden weight gain
☐ Restlessness and anxiety
☐ Change in mental status
☐ Intake greater than output, oliguria, specific gravity changes
☐ Shortness of breath, dyspnea, orthopnea
☐ Abnormal breath sounds (crackles, rales), change in respiratory pattern
☐ Pulmonary congestion by chest x-ray examination
☐ Blood pressure, venous pressure, pulmonary artery pressure changes
☐ Jugular vein distention; positive hepatojugular reflex, S_3 heart sound
☐ Hemoglobin and hematocrit decreased
☐ Electrolytes altered, azotemia

ETIOLOGICAL OR RELATED FACTORS
☐ Compromised regulatory mechanisms
☐ Excess fluid or sodium intake

[1]If diagnosed, refer for medical evaluation.

NOTES

High Risk for Impaired Skin Integrity *or* High Risk for Skin Breakdown

DEFINITION
☐ Presence of risk factors for skin ulceration, particularly over bony prominences

DEFINING CHARACTERISTICS
☐ Reddened skin area (especially over bony prominences)
☐ Verbalized pain or discomfort in local area (especially over bony prominences)
☐ Presence of shearing forces, pressure, friction (restraints, casts)
☐ Physical immobilization
☐ Excretions/secretions on skin
☐ Altered sensation, consciousness
☐ Lack of position change for greater than 1½ to 2 hours
☐ Alterations in nutritional state (obesity, emaciation, less than required protein intake, ascorbic acid deficiency)
☐ Altered metabolic state, anemia
☐ Altered circulation, edema, arteriosclerosis
☐ Psychogenic factors
☐ High humidity, environmental temperature
☐ Hypo-hyperthermia
☐ Medication (producing cellular breakdown)
☐ Altered pigmentation
☐ Decreased fatty tissue, skeletal prominence
☐ Alteration in skin turgor (change in elasticity)
☐ Immunologic factors
☐ Chemical substances on skin
☐ Radiation

NOTES

Impaired Skin Integrity

DEFINITION
- ☐ Break in skin integrity (if associated with bedrest or sitting condition, use Decubitus Ulcer).

DEFINING CHARACTERISTICS
- ☐ Disruption of skin surface
- ☐ Destruction of skin layers
- ☐ Invasion of body structures

ETIOLOGICAL OR RELATED FACTORS
- ☐ Altered circulation, metabolic state
- ☐ Hyper- or hypothermia
- ☐ Physical immobilization
- ☐ Humidity
- ☐ Alteration in turgor (elasticity)
- ☐ Altered nutritional status (obesity, emaciation)
- ☐ Altered sensation, pigmentation
- ☐ Immunological deficit
- ☐ Medication
- ☐ Developmental factors
- ☐ Psychogenic factors

NOTES

Pressure Ulcer (Specify Stage)

DEFINITION

☐ Break in skin integrity usually over bony prominences associated with lying or sitting for prolonged periods

DEFINING CHARACTERISTICS

☐ Ulceration (disruption of skin surface, usually over bony prominences)

☐ Verbalization of pain, discomfort, or numbness over bony prominence without exterior skin destruction (deep decubitus)

Stage I: Reddened area, no break in skin (see Potential Skin Breakdown)

Stage II: Reddened area; small ulceration

Stage III: Deep ulceration with drainage; no necrosis

Stage IV: Deep ulceration; necrotic area*

ETIOLOGICAL OR RELATED FACTORS

☐ Prolonged pressure
☐ Friction, shear injury
☐ Immobility
☐ Incontinence
☐ Undernutrition (protein, vitamin C)
☐ Sensory-motor loss
☐ Cognitive impairment

*Adapted from Michigan Nurses' Association, CURN Project: *Preventing decubitus ulcers*, New York, 1981. Grune & Stratton.

NOTES

Impaired Tissue Integrity (Specify Type)

DEFINITION

☐ A state in which an individual experiences damage to mucous membrane or to corneal, integumentary, or subcutaneous tissue

DEFINING CHARACTERISTICS

☐ *Damaged or destroyed tissue (cornea, mucous membrane, integumentary, or subcutaneous)

ETIOLOGICAL OR RELATED FACTORS

☐ Altered circulation
☐ Nutritional deficit/excess
☐ Fluid deficit/excess
☐ Knowledge deficit
☐ Impaired physical mobility
☐ Irritants:
  Chemical (body excretions, secretions, medications)
  Thermal (temperature extremes)
  Mechanical (pressure, shear, friction)
  Radiation (including therapeutic radiation)

NOTES

High Risk for Altered Body Temperature

DEFINITION

☐ The state in which the individual is at risk for failure to maintain body temperature within normal range

DEFINING CHARACTERISTICS (RISK FACTORS)

☐ Extremes of age
☐ Extremes of weight
☐ Exposure to cold/cool or warm/hot environments
☐ Dehydration
☐ Inactivity or vigorous activity
☐ Medications causing vasoconstriction/vasodilation
☐ Altered metabolic rate
☐ Sedation
☐ Inappropriate clothing for environmental temperature
☐ Illness or trauma affecting temperature regulation

NOTES

Ineffective Thermoregulation

DEFINITION
□ The state in which the individual's temperature fluctuates between hypothermia and hyperthermia

DEFINING CHARACTERISTICS
□ *Fluctuations in body temperature above or below the normal range
□ *(See defining characteristics of Hypothermia and Hyperthermia)

ETIOLOGICAL OR RELATED FACTORS
□ Trauma or illness
□ Immaturity
□ Aging
□ Fluctuating environmental temperature

NOTES

Hyperthermia

DEFINITION
☐ A state in which an individual's body temperature is elevated above his/her normal range

DEFINING CHARACTERISTICS
☐ *Increase in body temperature above normal range
☐ Flushed skin
☐ Skin warm to touch
☐ Increased respiratory rate
☐ Tachycardia
☐ Seizures/convulsions

ETIOLOGICAL OR RELATED FACTORS
☐ Exposure to hot environment
☐ Vigorous activity
☐ Medications/anesthesia
☐ Inappropriate clothing
☐ Increased metabolic rate
☐ Illness or trauma
☐ Dehydration
☐ Inability/decreased ability to perspire

NOTES

Hypothermia

DEFINITION
☐   Body temperature reduced below normal range

DEFINING CHARACTERISTICS
☐   Reduction in body temperature below normal range
☐   Shivering (mild)
☐   Cool skin; pallor (moderate); piloerection
☐   Slow capillary refill
☐   Tachycardia; cyanotic nail beds
☐   Hypertension

ETIOLOGICAL OR RELATED FACTORS
☐   Exposure to cool or cold environment
☐   Illness or trauma
☐   Inability or decreased ability to shiver
☐   Malnutrition; decreased metabolic rate; inactivity; aging
☐   Vasodilation; evaporation from skin in cool environment
☐   Damage to hypothalamus

NOTES

ELIMINATION PATTERN

NOTES

Constipation *or Intermittent Constipation Pattern*

DEFINITION
☐ Periodic episodes of hard, dry stools or absence of stools not associated with a pathological state

DEFINING CHARACTERISTICS
☐ *Frequency less than usual pattern
☐ *Hard formed stools, decreased quantity
☐ *Palpable mass
☐ *Reported feeling of pressure in rectum
☐ *Reported feeling of abdominal or rectal fullness
☐ *Straining at stool
☐ *Abdominal pain, cramps
☐ Appetite impairment
☐ Back pain
☐ Headache
☐ Interference with daily living
☐ Use of laxatives
☐ Nausea

ETIOLOGICAL OR RELATED FACTORS
☐ Low roughage diet
☐ Low fluid intake
☐ Decreased activity level
☐ Absence of routines (time)
☐ Routine use of enemas, laxatives

NOTES

Colonic Constipation

DEFINITION
- ☐ Pattern of elimination characterized by hard, dry stool which results from a delay in passage of food residue

DEFINING CHARACTERISTICS
- ☐ *Decreased frequency
- ☐ *Hard, dry stool
- ☐ Straining at stool
- ☐ Painful defecation
- ☐ Abdominal distention
- ☐ Palpable mass
- ☐ Rectal pressure
- ☐ Headache, appetite impairment
- ☐ Abdominal pain

ETIOLOGICAL OR RELATED FACTORS
- ☐ Less than adequate fluid intake
- ☐ Less than adequate dietary intake
- ☐ Less than adequate fiber
- ☐ Less than adequate physical activity, or immobility
- ☐ Chronic use of medication (laxatives) and enemas
- ☐ Lack of privacy
- ☐ Emotional disturbances; stress
- ☐ Change in daily routine
- ☐ Metabolic problems (e.g., hypothyroidism, hypocalcemia, hypokalemia)

NOTES

Perceived Constipation

DEFINITION
☐ Self-diagnosis of constipation and ensuring daily bowel
   movement through abuse of laxatives, enemas, and/or
   suppositories

DEFINING CHARACTERISTICS
☐ *Expectation of a daily bowel movement with the resulting
   overuse of laxatives, enemas, and/or suppositories
☐ Expected passage of stool at same time every day

ETIOLOGICAL OR RELATED FACTORS
☐ Cultural/family health beliefs
☐ Faulty appraisal
☐ Impaired thought processes

NOTES

Diarrhea

DEFINITION
- Frequent passage of loose, fluid, unformed stools not associated with a pathological state

DEFINING CHARACTERISTICS
- *Loose, fluid stools
- *Abdominal pain, discomfort
- *Cramping
- *Frequent bowel movements
- *Increased frequency of bowel sounds
- *Urgency
- Change in color of stools

ETIOLOGICAL OR RELATED FACTORS
- Food intolerance

NOTES

Bowel Incontinence

DEFINITION

☐   Involuntary passage of stool

DEFINING CHARACTERISTICS

☐   Involuntary passage of stool

ETIOLOGICAL OR RELATED FACTORS

☐   Loss of sphincter control
☐   Cognitive/perceptual impairment

NOTES

Altered Urinary Elimination Pattern[1,2]

DEFINITION

☐ Disturbance in pattern of urine elimination

DEFINING CHARACTERISTICS

☐ Dysuria
☐ Frequency
☐ Hesitancy
☐ Nocturia
☐ Retention
☐ Urgency
☐ Incontinence

[1]If diagnosed, refer for medical evaluation.
[2]See also Incontinence, pages 145-153 and retention, page 155.

NOTES

Functional Incontinence

DEFINITION

☐ The state in which an individual experiences an involuntary, unpredictable passage of urine

DEFINING CHARACTERISTICS

☐ *Urge to void or bladder contractions sufficiently strong to result in loss of urine before reaching an appropriate receptacle

ETIOLOGICAL OR RELATED FACTORS

☐ Altered environment
☐ Sensory deficits
☐ Cognitive deficits
☐ Mobility deficits

NOTES

Reflex Incontinence

DEFINITION
☐ The state in which an individual experiences an involuntary loss of urine, occurring at somewhat predictable intervals when a specific bladder volume is reached

DEFINING CHARACTERISTICS
☐ *No awareness of bladder filling
☐ *No urge to void or feelings of bladder fullness
☐ *Uninhibited bladder contraction/spasm at regular intervals

ETIOLOGICAL OR RELATED FACTORS
☐ Neurological impairment (e.g., spinal cord lesion which interferes with conduction of cerebral messages above the level of the reflex arc)

NOTES

Stress Incontinence

DEFINITION

☐ The state in which an individual experiences an involuntary loss of urine of less than 50 ml occurring with increased abdominal pressure

DEFINING CHARACTERISTICS

☐ *Reported or observed dribbling with increased abdominal pressure
☐ Urinary urgency
☐ Urinary frequency (more often than every 2 hours)

ETIOLOGICAL OR RELATED FACTORS

☐ Incompetent bladder outlet
☐ Age-related degenerative changes in pelvic muscles and structural supports
☐ Weak pelvic muscles and structural supports
☐ High intraabdominal pressure (e.g. obesity, gravid uterus)
☐ Overdistention between voidings

NOTES

Urge Incontinence

DEFINITION

□ The state in which an individual experiences involuntary passage of urine occurring soon after a strong sense of urgency to void

DEFINING CHARACTERISTICS

□ *Urinary urgency
□ *Frequency (voiding more often than every 2 hours)
□ *Bladder contracture/spasm
□ Nocturia (greater than 2 times per night)
□ Voiding in small amounts (less than 100 cc) or in large amounts (more than 550 cc)
□ Inability to reach toilet in time

ETIOLOGICAL OR RELATED FACTORS

□ Decreased bladder capacity (e.g., history of pelvic inflammatory disease, abdominal surgeries, indwelling urinary catheter)
□ Bladder spasm (irritation of bladder stretch receptors, e.g., bladder infection)
□ Alcohol
□ Caffeine
□ Increased fluids
□ Increased urine concentration
□ Overdistention of bladder

NOTES

Total Incontinence

DEFINITION

☐ The state in which an individual experiences a continuous and unpredictable loss of urine

DEFINING CHARACTERISTICS

☐ *Constant flow of urine at unpredictable times without distention or uninhibited bladder contractions/spasms
☐ *Unsuccessful incontinence refractory treatments
☐ *Nocturia
☐ Lack of perineal or bladder filling awareness
☐ Unawareness of incontinence

ETIOLOGICAL OR RELATED FACTORS

☐ Neuropathy (preventing transmission of reflex indicating bladder fullness)
☐ Neurological dysfunction (triggering micturition at unpredictable times)
☐ Independent contraction of detrusor reflex (resulting from surgery)
☐ Trauma (affecting spinal cord nerves)

NOTES

Urinary Retention[1]

DEFINITION

☐ The state in which the individual experiences incomplete
   emptying of the bladder

DEFINING CHARACTERISTICS

☐ *Bladder distention
☐ *Small, frequent voiding or absence of urine output
☐ Sensation of bladder fullness
☐ Dribbling
☐ Residual urine
☐ Dysuria
☐ Overflow incontinence

ETIOLOGICAL OR RELATED FACTORS

☐ High urethral pressure (caused by weak detrusor)
☐ Inhibition of reflex arc
☐ Strong sphinctor
☐ Blockage of urine

[1]If diagnosed, refer for medical evaluation.

NOTES

ACTIVITY-EXERCISE PATTERN

NOTES

High Risk for Activity Intolerance

DEFINITION
☐ Presence of risk factors for abnormal response to energy-consuming body movements

DEFINING CHARACTERISTICS (RISK FACTORS)
☐ Deconditioned status (prolonged bed rest, inactivity)
☐ Presence of circulatory or respiratory problems
☐ History of previous intolerance to activity
☐ Inexperience with the activity
☐ Intention, or need, to engage in energy-consuming body movement

NOTES

Activity Intolerance (Specify Level)

DEFINITION
☐ Abnormal responses to energy-consuming body movements involved in required or desired daily activities

DEFINING CHARACTERISTICS
☐ *Verbal report of fatigue or weakness
☐ External discomfort or dyspnea
☐ Abnormal responses to activity: heart rate, blood pressure, or electrocardiographic changes reflecting ischemia or arrhythmias
☐ Level 1: Walk, regular pace, on level indefinitely; one flight or more but more short of breath than normally
☐ Level II: Walk one city block 500 feet on level; climb one flight slowly without stopping
☐ Level III: Walk no more than 50 feet on level without stopping; unable to climb one flight of stairs without stopping
☐ Level IV: Dyspnea and fatigue at rest

ETIOLOGICAL OR RELATED FACTORS (Consider if activity intolerance is cause of another problem)
☐ Bed rest, immobility
☐ Sedentary lifestyle
☐ Imbalance between oxygen supply and demand
☐ Generalized weakness

NOTES

Fatigue

DEFINITION

- Overwhelming, sustained sense of exhaustion and decreased capacity for physical and mental work

DEFINING CHARACTERISTICS

- Verbalization of an unremitting and overwhelming lack of energy
- Inability to maintain usual routines
- Perceived need for additional energy to accomplish routine tasks
- Increase in physical complaints
- Emotionally labile or irritable
- Impaired ability to concentrate; lethargic or listless
- Decreased performance; accident-prone
- Disinterest in surroundings/introspection
- Decreased libido

ETIOLOGICAL OR RELATED FACTORS

- Overwhelming psychological/emotional demands
- Increased energy requirements to perform activities of daily living
- Excessive social and/or role demands
- Discomfort
- Altered body chemistry (e.g., medications, drug withdrawal, chemotherapy); decreased/increased metabolic energy production

NOTES

Impaired Physical Mobility (Specify Level[1])

DEFINITION
Limitation of ability for independent movement within the environment

DEFINING CHARACTERISTICS
☐ Inability to purposefully move within the physical environment (bed mobility, transfer, ambulation)
☐ Limited active joint range of motion
☐ Decreased muscle strength, control, and/or mass
☐ Impaired coordination
☐ Imposed restrictions of movement (mechanical or medical protocol restrictions)

☐ Level I: Requires use of equipment or device
☐ Level II: Requires help from another person(s): assistance, supervision or teaching
☐ Level III: Requires help from another person(s) and equipment device
☐ Level IV: Is dependent and does not participate in movement

---

[1]Adapted from E. Jones, et al: *Patient classification for long term care: Users manual*, HEW Publication No. HRA-74-3107. Washington, D.C., 1974, Department of Health, Education, and Welfare, Health Resources Administration, Bureau of Health Services Research and Evaluation.

(Continued)

NOTES

Impaired Physical Mobility (Specify Level) *Continued*

ETIOLOGICAL OR RELATED FACTORS

☐ Intolerance to activity; decreased strength and endurance (Decreased Activity Tolerance)
☐ Pain; discomfort
☐ Uncompensated perceptual-cognitive impairment
☐ Uncompensated musculoskeletal impairment
☐ Uncompensated neuromuscular impairment
☐ Depression
☐ Severe anxiety

NOTES

High Risk for Disuse Syndrome

DEFINITION

☐ Presence of risk factors for deterioration of body systems as the result of prescribed or unavoidable musculoskeletal inactivity

DEFINING CHARACTERISTICS (RISK FACTORS)

☐ Paralysis
☐ Mechanical immobilization
☐ Prescribed immobilization
☐ Severe pain
☐ Altered level of consciousness

NOTES

High Risk For Joint Contractures

DEFINITION
☐ Presence of risk factors for shortening of tendons at movable joints (back head, upper and lower extremities)

DEFINING CHARACTERISTICS (RISK FACTORS)
☐ Maintenance of joint flexion in upright, sitting, or recumbent posture for long periods of time
☐ Neuromuscular pathological condition associated with joint flexion (e.g., lack of voluntary postural muscle control, spasticity)
☐ Assumption of abnormal posture resulting from psychosocial factors or cognitive deficit

NOTES

Total Self-Care Deficit (Specify Level)

DEFINITION
□ Inability to complete feeding, bathing, toileting, dressing, grooming of self

DEFINING CHARACTERISTICS
□ Observation or valid report of inability to eat, bathe, toilet, dress, groom self independently (See defining characteristics for each deficit.)
□ Level I: Requires use of equipment or devices
□ Level II: Requires help from another person(s): assistance, supervision, teaching
□ Level III: Requires help from another person(s) *and* equipment or device
□ Level IV: Is dependent and does not participate in self-care

ETIOLOGICAL OR RELATED FACTORS
□ Intolerance to activity; decreased strength and endurance (Decreased activity tolerance)
□ Pain; discomfort
□ Uncompensated perceptual-cognitive impairment
□ Uncompensated neuromuscular impairment
□ Uncompensated musculoskeletal impairment
□ Severe anxiety
□ Depression

NOTES

Self-Bathing—Hygiene Deficit (Specify Level)

DEFINITION
☐ Inability to bathe body or body parts

DEFINING CHARACTERISTICS
☐ *Inability to wash body or body parts
☐ Inability to obtain or get to water source
☐ Inability to regulate temperature or flow

☐ Level I: Requires use of equipment or devices
☐ Level II: Requires help from another person(s): assistance, supervision, teaching
☐ Level III: Requires help from another person(s) and equipment or device
☐ Level IV: Is dependent and does not participate in self-bathing/hygiene

ETIOLOGICAL OR RELATED FACTORS
☐ Intolerance to activity; decreased strength and endurance (Decreased activity tolerance)
☐ Pain; discomfort
☐ Uncompensated perceptual-cognitive impairment
☐ Uncompensated neuromuscular impairment
☐ Uncompensated musculoskeletal impairment
☐ Severe anxiety
☐ Depression

NOTES

Self-Dressing—Grooming Deficit (Specify Level)

DEFINITION
- Inability to dress or groom self

DEFINING CHARACTERISTICS
- *Impaired ability to put on or take off necessary items of clothing
- Impaired ability to obtain or replace articles of clothing
- Impaired ability to fasten clothing
- Inability to maintain appearance at a satisfactory level

- Level I: Requires use of equipment or devices
- Level II: Requires help from another person(s): assistance, supervision, teaching
- Level III: Requires help from another person(s) and equipment or device
- Level IV: Is dependent and does not participate in self-dressing and grooming

ETIOLOGICAL OR RELATED FACTORS
- Intolerance to activity; decreased strength and endurance (Decreased activity tolerance)
- Pain; discomfort
- Uncompensated perceptual-cognitive impairment
- Uncompensated neuromuscular impairment
- Uncompensated musculoskeletal impairment
- Severe anxiety
- Depression

NOTES

Self-Feeding Deficit (Specify Level)

DEFINITION
☐ Inability to feed self when food available

DEFINING CHARACTERISTICS
☐ *Inability to bring food from a receptacle to the mouth
☐ Level I: Requires use of equipment or devices
☐ Level II: Requires help from another person(s): assistance, supervision, teaching
☐ Level III: Requires assistance or supervision from another person(s) and equipment or device
☐ Level IV: Is dependent and does not participate in self-feeding

ETIOLOGICAL OR RELATED FACTORS
☐ Intolerance to activity; decreased strength and endurance (Decreased activity tolerance)
☐ Pain; discomfort
☐ Uncompensated perceptual-cognitive impairment
☐ Uncompensated neuromuscular impairment
☐ Uncompensated musculoskeletal impairment
☐ Severe anxiety
☐ Depression

NOTES

Self-Toileting Deficit (Specify Level)

DEFINITION
□ Inability to toilet

DEFINING CHARACTERISTICS
□ *Unable to get to toilet or commode
□ *Unable to sit on or rise from toilet or commode
□ *Unable to manipulate clothing for toileting
□ *Unable to carry out proper toilet hygiene
□ Unable to flush toilet or empty commode
□ Level I: Requires use of equipment or devices
□ Level II: Requires help from another person(s): assistance, supervision, teaching
□ Level III: Requires help from another person(s) and equipment or device
□ Level IV: Is dependent and does not participate in self-toileting

ETIOLOGICAL OR RELATED FACTORS
□ Impaired transfer ability
□ Impaired mobility
□ Intolerance to activity; decreased strength and endurance (Decreased activity tolerance)
□ Pain; discomfort
□ Uncompensated perceptual-cognitive impairment
□ Uncompensated neuromuscular impairment
□ Uncompensated musculoskeletal impairment
□ Severe anxiety
□ Depression

NOTES

Altered Growth and Development: Self-Care Skills (Specify Level)[1]

DEFINITION

☐ Demonstrates deviations from age-group norms for self care skills

DEFINING CHARACTERISTICS

☐ *Delay or difficulty in performing self-care skills typical of age group/developmental level (eating, bathing/hygiene, toileting, dressing/grooming)
☐ Flat affect
☐ Listlessness
☐ Decreased responses

ETIOLOGICAL OR RELATED FACTORS

☐ Environmental and stimulation deficiencies
☐ Inadequate caretaking:
  Indifference
  Inconsistent responsiveness
  Multiple caretakers
☐ Separation (from significant others)
☐ Physical disability effects
☐ Prescribed dependence

[1]See p. 215 Altered Growth and Development, for accepted diagnosis.

NOTES

Diversional Activity Deficit

DEFINITION
☐ Decreased engagement in recreational or leisure activities

DEFINING CHARACTERISTICS
☐ Report of boredom
☐ Daytime napping
☐ Usual hobbies or activities cannot be undertaken (e.g., in hospital)
☐ Expressed wish for something to do, to read, etc.

ETIOLOGICAL OR RELATED FACTORS
☐ Long-term hospitalization — apathy
☐ Environmental lack of diversional activity
☐ Frequent lengthy treatments

NOTES

Impaired Home Maintenance Management (Mild, Moderate, Severe, Potential, Chronic)

DEFINITION

□ Inability to independently maintain a safe, growth-promoting immediate environment

DEFINING CHARACTERISTICS

□ *Household members express difficulty in maintaining their home in a comfortable fashion
□ *Household members describe outstanding debts or financial crises
□ *Unwashed or unavailable cooking equipment, clothes, or linen
□ *Overtaxed family members (e.g., exhausted, anxious family members)
□ *Repeated hygienic disorders, infestations, or infections
□ Household members request assistance with home maintenance
□ Disorderly surroundings
□ Accumulation of dirt, food wastes, or hygienic wastes
□ Offensive odors
□ Inappropriate household temperature
□ Lack of necessary equipment or aids
□ Presence of vermin or rodents

(Continued)

NOTES

Impaired Home Maintenance Management (Mild, Moderate, Severe, Potential, Chronic) *Continued*

ETIOLOGICAL OR RELATED FACTORS

- ☐ Individual/family member disease or injury
- ☐ Insufficient family organization/planning
- ☐ Insufficient finances
- ☐ Unfamiliarity with neighborhood resources
- ☐ Impaired cognitive or emotional functioning
- ☐ Knowledge deficit
- ☐ Lack of role modeling
- ☐ Inadequate support systems

NOTES

Dysfunctional Ventilatory Weaning Response (DVWR)

DEFINITION

☐ Inability to adjust to lowered levels of mechanical ventilator support, which interrupts and prolongs the weaning process (mild, moderate, severe)

DEFINING CHARACTERISTICS
Mild DVWR

Responds to lowered levels of mechanical ventilator support with:

☐ *Restlessness
☐ *Slight increase in respiratory rate from baseline
☐ Expression of increased need for oxygen; breathing discomfort; fatigue; warmth
☐ Queries about possible machine malfunction
☐ Increased concentration on breathing

Moderate DVWR

Responds to lowered levels of mechanical ventilator support with:

☐ *Slight increase from baseline blood pressure <20 mm Hg
☐ *Slight increase from baseline heart rate <20 beats/minute
☐ *Baseline increase in respiratory rate <5 breaths/minute
☐ Hypervigilance to activities
☐ Inability to respond to coaching
☐ Inability to cooperate
☐ Apprehension
☐ Diaphoresis
☐ Eye widening ("wide-eyed look")   *(Continued)*

NOTES

Dysfunctional Ventilatory Weaning Response (DVWR) *Continued*

- ☐ Decreased air entry on auscultation
- ☐ Color changes (pale, slight cyanosis)
- ☐ Slight respiratory accessory muscle use

Severe DVWR

Responds to lowered levels of mechanical ventilator support with:

- ☐ *Agitation
- ☐ *Deterioration in arterial blood gases from current baseline
- ☐ *Increase from baseline blood pressure >20 mm Hg
- ☐ *Increase from baseline heart rate >20 beats/minute
- ☐ *Respiratory rate increases significantly from baseline
- ☐ Profuse diaphoresis
- ☐ Full respiratory accessory muscle use
- ☐ Shallow, gasping breaths
- ☐ Paradoxical abdominal breathing
- ☐ Discoordinated breathing with the ventilator
- ☐ Decreased level of consciousness
- ☐ Adventitious breath sounds, audible airway secretions
- ☐ Cyanosis

ETIOLOGICAL OR RELATED FACTORS
Physical

- ☐ Ineffective airway clearance
- ☐ Sleep pattern disturbance
- ☐ Inadequate nutrition
- ☐ Uncontrolled pain or discomfort   *(Continued)*

NOTES

Dysfunctional Ventilatory Weaning Response (DVWR) *Continued*

Psychological

- ☐ Knowledge deficit (weaning process; patient role)
- ☐ Perceived inability to wean
- ☐ Decreased motivation
- ☐ Decreased self-esteem
- ☐ Anxiety: moderate, severe
- ☐ Fear
- ☐ Hopelessness
- ☐ Powerlessness
- ☐ Insufficient trust in the nurse

Situational

- ☐ Uncontrolled episodic energy demands/problems
- ☐ Inappropriate pacing of diminished ventilator support
- ☐ Inadequate social support
- ☐ Adverse environment (e.g., noisy, active environment; negative events in the room; low nurse-patient ratio; extended nurse absence from bedside; unfamiliar nursing staff)
- ☐ History of ventilator dependence >1 week
- ☐ History of multiple unsuccessful weaning attempts

NOTES

Inability to Sustain Spontaneous Ventilation[1]

DEFINITION

☐ Decreased energy/reserves resulting in an individual's inability to maintain breathing adequate to support life

DEFINING CHARACTERISTICS

☐ *Dyspnea
☐ *Increased metabolic rate
☐ Increased restlessness
☐ Apprehension
☐ Increased use of accessory muscles
☐ Decreased tidal volume
☐ Increased heart rate
☐ Decreased Po_2
☐ Increased Pco_2
☐ Decreased Sao_2
☐ Decreased cooperation

ETIOLOGICAL OR RELATED FACTORS

☐ Metabolic factors (specify)
☐ Respiratory muscle fatigue

[1]If diagnosed, refer for immediate medical evaluation.

NOTES

Ineffective Airway Clearance

DEFINITION
☐   Inability to effectively clear secretions or obstruction from
    respiratory tract

DEFINING CHARACTERISTICS
☐   Abnormal breath sounds (rales, crackles, rhonchi, wheezes)
☐   Cough (effective/ineffective; with or without sputum)
☐   Change in rate or depth of respiration
☐   Tachypnea (rate increase)
☐   Dyspnea at rest or on exertion
☐   Cyanosis

ETIOLOGICAL OR RELATED FACTORS
☐   Excess thick secretions
☐   Decreased energy/fatigue
☐   Altered level of consciousness
☐   Pain
☐   Obstruction
☐   Tracheobronchial infection
☐   Trauma
☐   Perceptual/cognitive impairment

NOTES

Ineffective Breathing Pattern[1]

DEFINITION
☐ Respiration (respiratory compensations) inadequate to maintain sufficient oxygen supply for cellular requirements

DEFINING CHARACTERISTICS
☐ Dyspnea, shortness of breath
☐ Use of accessory muscles
☐ Altered chest excursion
☐ Tachypnea
☐ Cough
☐ Nasal flaring
☐ Respiratory depth changes
☐ Assumption of three-point position
☐ Pursed-lip breathing/prolonged expiratory phase
☐ Increased anteroposterior diameter
☐ Fremitus
☐ Abnormal arterial blood gases
☐ Cyanosis

ETIOLOGICAL OR RELATED FACTORS
☐ Neuromuscular impairment
☐ Musculoskeletal impairment
☐ Perceptual/cognitive impairment
☐ Anxiety
☐ Decreased energy/fatigue
☐ Pain

[1]If diagnosed, refer for medical evaluation.

NOTES

Impaired Gas Exchange[1]

DEFINITION
☐ Disturbance in oxygen or carbon dioxide exchange in lungs
   or at cellular level

DEFINING CHARACTERISTICS
☐ Confusion
☐ Somnolence
☐ Restlessness
☐ Irritability
☐ Inability to move secretions
☐ Hypercapnea
☐ Hypoxia

ETIOLOGICAL OR RELATED FACTORS
☐ Ventilation-perfusion imbalance

[1]If diagnosed, refer for medical evaluation.

NOTES

Decreased Cardiac Output[1]

DEFINITION
☐ Presence of indicators of lowered cardiac output

DEFINING CHARACTERISTICS
☐ *Variations in blood pressure readings
☐ *Jugular vein distention
☐ *Decreased peripheral pulses
☐ *Arrythmia
☐ *Color changes in skin and mucous membranes
☐ *Cold, clammy skin
☐ *Fatigue
☐ *Oliguria
☐ *Rales
☐ *Dyspnea
☐ *Orthopnea
☐ *Restlessness
☐ Change in mental status
☐ Syncope, vertigo
☐ Cough, frothy sputum
☐ Edema
☐ Gallop rhythm
☐ Weakness

ETIOLOGICAL OR RELATED FACTORS
☐ (To be identified)

[1]If diagnosed, refer for medical evaluation.

NOTES

Altered Tissue Perfusion (Specify)[1]

DEFINITION
- Chronic deficit in blood supply to a part relative to metabolic needs (cerebral, cardiopulmonary, renal, gastrointestinal, peripheral)

DEFINING CHARACTERISTICS
- *Cold extremities
- *Extremities blue or purple when dependent; pale on elevation and color does not return on lowering leg
- *Diminished arterial pulsations
- Shiny skin surfaces
- Lack of lanugo hair
- Round scars covered with atrophied skin
- Gangrene
- Slow-growing, dry, thick, brittle nails
- Claudication
- Blood pressure changes in extremities
- Bruits
- Slow healing of lesions; gangrene

ETIOLOGICAL OR RELATED FACTORS
- Interruption of arterial flow
- Interruption of venous flow
- Exchange problems
- Hypovolemia
- Hypervolemia

[1]If diagnosed, refer for medical evaluation.

NOTES

Dysreflexia[1]

DEFINITION

☐ The state in which an individual with a spinal cord injury at T7 or above experiences a life-threatening uninhibited sympathetic response of the nervous system to a noxious stimulus

DEFINING CHARACTERISTICS

☐ Individual with spinal cord injury (T7 or above)
☐ Paroxysmal hypertension (sudden, periodic elevated blood pressure; systolic pressure over 140 mm Hg and diastolic above 90 mm Hg)
☐ Bradycardia or tachycardia (pulse rate of less than 60 or over 100 beats per minute)
☐ Diaphoresis (above the injury)
☐ Red splotches on skin (above the injury)
☐ Headache (a diffuse pain in different portions of the head; not confined to any nerve distribution area)
☐ Paresthesia
☐ Chilling; pilomotor reflex (gooseflesh formation when skin is cooled)
☐ Conjunctival congestion
☐ Blurred vision
☐ Horner's syndrome (contraction of the pupil, partial ptosis of the eyelid, enophthalmos, sometimes loss of sweating over the affected side of the face)
☐ Chest pain

[1]Preventive care can be organized under the diagnosis High Risk for Dysreflexia.

NOTES

Dysreflexia *Continued*

- ☐ Metallic taste in mouth
- ☐ Nasal congestion

ETIOLOGICAL OR RELATED FACTORS

- ☐ Bladder distention
- ☐ Bowel distention
- ☐ Skin irritation

NOTES

High Risk for Peripheral Neurovascular Dysfunction[1]

DEFINITION

☐ Presence of risk factors for disruption in circulation, sensation, or motion of an extremity

RISK FACTORS

☐ Immobilization
☐ Mechanical compression (e.g., tourniquet, cast/brace, dressing/restraint)
☐ Orthopaedic surgery
☐ Trauma
☐ Burns
☐ Vascular obstruction
☐ Fractures

[1]Diagnosis encompasses three foci (nutrient supply to tissues, sensation, and motion), thus it can be viewed as a potentially dysfunctional nutritional/metabolic, perceptual, or activity pattern.

NOTES

Altered Growth and Development

DEFINITION

☐ The state in which an individual demonstrates deviations in norms from his/her age group

DEFINING CHARACTERISTICS

☐ *Delay or difficulty in performing skills (motor, social, or expressive) typical of age group
☐ *Altered physical growth
☐ *Inability to perform self-care or self-control activities appropriate for age

ETIOLOGICAL OR RELATED FACTORS

☐ Inadequate caretaking:
   Indifference
   Inconsistent responsiveness
   Multiple caretakers
☐ Separation (from significant others)
☐ Environmental and stimulation deficiencies
☐ Physical disability effects
☐ Prescribed dependence

NOTES

SLEEP-REST PATTERN

NOTES

Sleep-Pattern Disturbance

DEFINITION
☐ Disruption of sleep time causing discomfort or interference with desired life activities

DEFINING CHARACTERISTICS
☐ *Verbal complaints of difficulty falling asleep (sleep onset)
☐ *Early awakening
☐ *Interrupted sleep
☐ *Sleep pattern reversal
☐ *Verbal complaints of not feeling well rested
☐ Reduction in performance (work, school, home)
☐ Increasing irritability
☐ Restlessness
☐ Disorientation (progressive)
☐ Lethargy
☐ Listlessness
☐ Mild, fleeting nystagmus
☐ Slight hand tremor
☐ Ptosis of eyelids
☐ Expressionless face
☐ Thick speech with mispronunciation and incorrect words
☐ Dark circles under eyes
☐ Frequent yawning
☐ Changes in posture

(Continued)

NOTES

Sleep-Pattern Disturbance *Continued*

ETIOLOGICAL OR RELATED FACTORS

- ☐ Physical discomfort (specify)
- ☐ Personal stress
- ☐ Family stress
- ☐ Environmental or habit changes
- ☐ Daytime boredom, inactivity
- ☐ Fear (specify)

NOTES

COGNITIVE-PERCEPTUAL PATTERN

NOTES

Pain

DEFINITION

☐ Verbal report and presence of indicators of severe discomfort (pain)

DEFINING CHARACTERISTICS

☐ Communication (verbal or coded) of pain descriptors
☐ Guarding behavior—protective
☐ Self-focusing
☐ Narrowed focus (altered time perception, withdrawal from social contact, impaired thought process)
☐ Distraction behavior (moaning, crying, pacing, seeking out other people and/or activities, restless)
☐ Facial mask of pain (eyes lack luster, "beaten look," fixed or scattered movement, grimace)
☐ Alteration in muscle tone (may span from listless to rigid)
☐ Autonomic responses not seen in chronic, stable pain (diaphoresis, blood pressure and pulse rate change, pupillary dilation, increased or decreased respiratory rate)

ETIOLOGICAL OR RELATED FACTORS

☐ Knowledge deficit (pain management techniques)
☐ Injuring agents (biological, chemical, physical, psychological)

NOTES

Chronic Pain

DEFINITION

☐ A state in which the individual experiences pain that continues for more than 6 months in duration

DEFINING CHARACTERISTICS

☐ *Verbal report or observed evidence of pain experienced for more than 6 months
☐ Facial masks (of pain)
☐ Guarded movement
☐ Fear of reinjury
☐ Physical and social withdrawal
☐ Altered ability to continue previous activities
☐ Anorexia
☐ Weight changes
☐ Changes in sleep pattern

ETIOLOGICAL OR RELATED FACTORS

☐ Chronic physical/psychosocial disability

NOTES

Pain Self-Management Deficit (Acute, Chronic)

DEFINITION

☐ Episodes of severe discomfort (pain) related to lack of knowledge or skill in application of pain self-management techniques (pain medication requests, timing, positioning, distraction, etc.)

DEFINING CHARACTERISTICS

☐ *Communication (verbal or coded) of pain descriptors
☐ *Delayed requests for medication, lack of use of positioning, distraction, etc.
☐ Guarding behavior—protective
☐ Self-focusing
☐ Narrowed focus of attention as evidenced by altered time perception, withdrawal from social contact, impaired thought process
☐ Distraction behavior as evidenced by moaning, crying, pacing, restlessness
☐ Facial mask of pain as evidenced by lackluster eyes, fixed or scattered movement, grimace
☐ Alteration in muscle tone (listless to rigid)

ETIOLOGICAL OR RELATED FACTORS

☐ Insufficient knowledge (Pain Management Techniques)

NOTES

Uncompensated Sensory Deficit (Specify)

DEFINITION

☐ Uncompensated loss of acuity, or absence, of vision, hearing, touch, smell, or kinesthesia

DEFINING CHARACTERISTICS

Vision
☐ Inability to read newsprint, or identify objects and persons
Hearing
☐ Inability to identify whispered sounds or normally voiced words
Touch
☐ Inability to discriminate various qualities or tactile sensations or absence of tactile perception
Smell
☐ Inability to identify odors
Kinesthesia
☐ Inability to identify extent, direction or weight of movement of body or body part

ETIOLOGICAL OR RELATED FACTORS

☐ (May be an etiology of other problems)

NOTES

Sensory-Perceptual Alteration: Input Deficit *or Sensory Deprivation*

DEFINITION
☐ Reduced environmental and social stimuli relative to habitual (or basic orienting) level

DEFINING CHARACTERISTICS
☐ Alert with periodic disorientation, general confusion, or nocturnal confusion
☐ Hallucinations
☐ Apathy
☐ Auditory, visual, reality-orienting, or time-orienting input reduced or absent
☐ Limited proprioceptive input
☐ Presence of uncompensated visual or hearing deficits

ETIOLOGICAL OR RELATED FACTORS
☐ Isolation (restricted environment)
☐ Therapeutic environmental restriction (specify: isolation, intensive care, bed rest, traction, confining illness, incubator)
☐ Socially restricted environment (specify: institutionalization, homebound, age-debilitation, infant deprivation)
☐ Uncompensated visual or hearing deficit
☐ Impaired communication

NOTES

Sensory-Perceptual Alteration: Input Excess *or Sensory Overload*

DEFINITION

☐ Environmental stimuli greater than habitual level of input and/or monotonous environmental stimuli

DEFINING CHARACTERISTICS

☐ Irritability, anxiety
☐ Restlessness
☐ Disorientation (periodic or general)
☐ Sleeplessness
☐ Reduction in problem-solving ability, work performance
☐ Complaints of fatigue
☐ Increased muscle tension
☐ Uninterrupted and/or unchanging stimuli (motor, monitor, light, voices)
☐ Amount or complexity of stimuli exceeds cognitive capabilities to handle sensory input

ETIOLOGICAL OR RELATED FACTORS

☐ Environmental complexity/monotony

NOTES

Unilateral Neglect

DEFINITION

☐ The state in which an individual is perceptually unaware of and inattentive to one side of the body

DEFINING CHARACTERISTICS

☐ *Consistent inattention to stimuli on the affected side
☐ Inadequate self-care (of affected side)
☐ Lack of positioning and/or safety precautions in regard to the affected side
☐ Does not look toward affected side
☐ Leaves food on plate on the affected side

ETIOLOGICAL OR RELATED FACTORS

☐ Effects of disturbed perceptual abilities (e.g., hemianopsia; one-sided blindness; neurological illness or trauma)

NOTES

Knowledge Deficit (Specify)

DEFINITION
- ☐ Inability to state or explain information or demonstrate a required skill related to disease management procedures, practices, and/or self-care–health management

DEFINING CHARACTERISTICS
- ☐ Verbalizations indicate less than adequate recall of information or inadequate understanding, misinterpretation, or misconception
- ☐ Inaccurate follow-through of previous instruction
- ☐ Inadequate performance of a test or demonstration of a skill
- ☐ Inappropriate or exaggerated behaviors (e.g., hysterical, hostile, agitated, apathetic)

ETIOLOGICAL OR RELATED FACTORS
- ☐ Low readiness for reception of information (e.g., anxiety)
- ☐ Lack of interest or motivation to learn
- ☐ Cognitive limitations (intellectual)
- ☐ Uncompensated memory loss
- ☐ Inability to use materials or information resources (e.g., cultural-language differences)
- ☐ Unfamiliarity with information resources

NOTES

Impaired Thought Processes

DEFINITION

☐ Discrepancy between manifested cognitive operations and expected cognitive operations for chronological age

DEFINING CHARACTERISTICS

☐ Impaired attention span, distractibility
☐ Inappropriate behavior; nonreality-based thinking
☐ Impaired recall ability
☐ Impaired ability to grasp ideas (conceptualize) or order ideas (reason and reflection)
☐ Impaired perception, judgment, decision making
☐ Increased self-concern (egocentricity)
☐ Hypo- or hypervigilance

ETIOLOGICAL OR RELATED FACTORS

☐ Developmental lag
☐ Sensory overload (environmental complexity)

NOTES

Uncompensated Short-Term Memory Deficit

DEFINITION
☐ Impaired ability to recall recent or current events and activities

DEFINING CHARACTERISTICS
☐ Frequent episodes of inability to recall recent events, information received, and/or activities
☐ Lack of understanding and problem solving deficit in short-term recall (minutes, hours)
☐ Begins an activity and unable to recall intention seconds or minutes later
☐ Inability to recall previously learned activities, names, places, etc.

ETIOLOGICAL OR RELATED FACTORS
☐ (May be of other problems)

NOTES

High Risk for Cognitive Impairment

DEFINITION

☐ At high risk for impairment in memory, reasoning ability, judgment, and decision making

DEFINING CHARACTERISTICS (RISK FACTORS)

☐ Low self-initiative in providing cognitive stimulation
☐ Confinement to environment low in cognitive (perceptual, problem solving, decision making) stimulation
☐ Hearing and/or vision deficit
☐ Borderline neurophysiological pathological condition
☐ Receiving tranquilizers, sedatives

NOTES

Decisional Conflict (Specify)

DEFINITION

☐ State of uncertainty about course of action to be taken when choice among competing actions involves risk, loss, or challenge to personal life values (Specify focus of conflict, e.g., surgery, therapy, abortion, divorce, or other life events)

DEFINING CHARACTERISTICS

☐ Verbalized uncertainty about choices
☐ Verbalization of undesired consequences of alternative actions being considered
☐ Delayed decision making or vacillation between alternative choices
☐ Verbalized feeling of distress while attempting a decision
☐ Questioning personal values and beliefs while attempting a decision
☐ Self-focusing
☐ Physical signs of distress or tension (increased heart rate, increased muscle tension, restlessness, etc.)

ETIOLOGICAL OR RELATED FACTORS

☐ Unclear personal values/beliefs
☐ Perceived threat to value system
☐ Lack of experience or interference with decision making
☐ Lack of relevant information; multiple/divergent information sources
☐ Support system deficit

NOTES

SELF-PERCEPTION–
SELF-CONCEPT PATTERN

NOTES

Fear (Specify Focus)

DEFINITION
☐ Feeling of dread related to an identifiable source which is perceived as a threat or danger to the self

DEFINING CHARACTERISTICS
☐ Describes, with or without assistance, the focus of perceived threat or danger (potential, actual, or imagined)
☐ Feelings of dread, nervousness, or concern about a threatening event, person, object
☐ Verbalized expectation of danger to the self
☐ Increased questioning or information-seeking
☐ Restlessness
☐ Voice tremors, pitch changes
☐ Increase in quantity of verbalization
☐ Increased rate of verbalization
☐ Hand tremor
☐ Increased muscle tension
☐ Narrowing focus of attention progressing to fixed
☐ Diaphoresis
☐ Increased heart rate
☐ Increased respiratory rate

ETIOLOGICAL OR RELATED FACTORS
☐ Knowledge deficit
☐ Perceived inability to control event

NOTES

Anxiety

DEFINITION

☐ Vague, uneasy feeling, the source of which is often nonspecific or unknown to the individual

DEFINING CHARACTERISTICS

☐ Verbalizes apprehension, uncertainty, fear, distress, worry
☐ Verbalizes painful and persistent feelings of increased helplessness, inadequacy, regret
☐ Expresses concern (change in life events)
☐ Fear of unspecified consequences
☐ Overexcited, rattled, jittery, scared
☐ Restlessness, focus on self, insomnia, increased perspiration
☐ Increased wariness, glancing about, poor eye contact, facial tension, voice quivering
☐ Increased tension, foot shuffling, hand/arm movements, trembling, hand tremor, shakiness

ETIOLOGICAL OR RELATED FACTORS

☐ Perceived threat to self-concept, health status, socioeconomic status, role functioning, interaction patterns, or environment
☐ Perceived threat of death
☐ Unconscious conflict (essential values, life goals)
☐ Unmet needs (specify)
☐ Interpersonal transmission/contagion

NOTES

Mild Anxiety

DEFINITION

☐ Increased level of arousal associated with expectation of a threat (unfocused) to the self or significant relationships

DEFINING CHARACTERISTICS

☐ Verbalizes feelings of increased arousal and concern
☐ Increased questioning
☐ Restlessness
☐ Increased awareness
☐ Increased attending
☐ Mild restlessness

ETIOLOGICAL OR RELATED FACTORS

☐ (To be identified)

NOTES

Moderate Anxiety

DEFINITION
☐ Increased level of arousal associated with expectation of a threat (unfocused) to the self or significant relationships

DEFINING CHARACTERISTICS
☐ Expressed feelings of unfocused apprehension, nervousness, or concern
☐ Verbalizes expectation of danger
☐ Voice tremors, pitch changes
☐ Restlessness
☐ Increased rate of verbalization
☐ Increase in quantity of verbalization
☐ Pacing
☐ Hand tremor
☐ Increased muscle tension
☐ Narrowing focus of attention
☐ Diaphoresis
☐ Increased heart rate
☐ Increased respiratory rate
☐ Sleep or eating disturbances

ETIOLOGICAL OR RELATED FACTORS
☐ Separation (use separation anxiety)

NOTES

Severe Anxiety (Panic)

DEFINITION

☐ Increased level of arousal associated with expectation of a threat to the self or to significant relationships

DEFINING CHARACTERISTICS

☐ Expressed feelings of unfocused, severe dread; apprehension; nervousness; or concern
☐ Inappropriate verbalization or absence of verbalization
☐ Purposeless activity or immobilization
☐ Perceptual focus scattered, fixed, or inability to focus on reality
☐ Increased heart rate
☐ Hyperventilation
☐ Diaphoresis
☐ Increased muscle tension
☐ Dilated pupils
☐ Pallor

ETIOLOGICAL OR RELATED FACTORS

☐ (To be identified)

NOTES

Anticipatory Anxiety (Mild, Moderate, Severe)

DEFINITION

☐ Increased level of arousal associated with a perceived future threat (unfocused) to the self or significant relationships

DEFINING CHARACTERISTICS

☐ Indicators of anxiety (see Anxiety)
☐ Future/impending event perceived as a threat to physical or psychosocial self (unfocused)

ETIOLOGICAL OR RELATED FACTORS

☐ (To be identified)

NOTES

Reactive Depression (Situational)

DEFINITION
☐ Acute decrease in self-esteem or worth related to a threat to self-competency

DEFINING CHARACTERISTICS
☐ Expressions of hopelessness, despair
☐ Inability to concentrate on reading, writing, conversation
☐ Change (usually decrease) in physical activities, eating, sleeping (early morning awakening), sexual activity
☐ Continual questioning of self-worth (self-esteem)
☐ Feeling of failure (real or imagined)
☐ Withdrawal from others to avoid possible rejection (real or imagined)
☐ Threats or attempts to commit suicide
☐ Suspicion and sensitivity to words and actions of others related to general lack of trust of others
☐ Misdirected anger (toward self)
☐ General irritability
☐ Guilt feelings
☐ Extreme dependency on others with related feelings of helplessness and anger

ETIOLOGICAL OR RELATED FACTORS
☐ Perceived powerlessness

NOTES

Hopelessness

DEFINITION
- A subjective state in which an individual sees limited or no alternatives or personal choices available and is unable to mobilize energy on own behalf

DEFINING CHARACTERISTICS
- *Passivity
- *Decreased verbalization
- *Decreased affect
- *Verbalization of despondent or hopeless content (e.g., "I can't," sighing)
- Lack of initiative
- Decreased response to stimuli
- Lack of involvement in care/passively allowing care
- Turning away from speaker
- Closing eyes
- Shrugging in response to speaker
- Decreased appetite
- Increased sleep

ETIOLOGICAL OR RELATED FACTORS
- Prolonged activity restriction (creating isolation)
- Failing or deteriorating physiologic condition
- Long-term stress
- Abandonment
- Loss of belief (transcendent values/God)

NOTES

Powerlessness (Severe, Moderate, Low)

DEFINITION
- Perceived lack of control over a situation and that own actions will not significantly effect an outcome

DEFINING CHARACTERISTICS
Severe
- Verbalization of having no control (situation, outcome, or self-care)
- Depression over physical deterioration (occurring despite compliance with regimes)
- Apathy

Moderate
- Nonparticipation in care of decision making when opportunities provided
- Expressed dissatisfaction or frustration over inability to perform previous tasks/activities
- Expressed doubt regarding role performance
- Passivity
- Does not monitor progress, seek information regarding care, or defend self-care practices when challenged
- Dependence on others that may result in irritability, resentment, anger, and guilt
- Reluctance to express true feelings fearing alienation from caregivers

Low Passivity
- Expressed uncertainty about fluctuating energy levels

(Continued)

NOTES

Powerlessness (Severe, Moderate, Low)

Continued

ETIOLOGICAL OR RELATED FACTORS

☐ Illness-related regime
☐ Health care environment
☐ Interpersonal interaction
☐ Lifestyle of helplessness

NOTES

Self-Esteem Disturbance

DEFINITION
☐ Negative self-evaluation/feelings about self or self-capabilities which may be directly or indirectly expressed

DEFINING CHARACTERISTICS
☐ Self-negating verbalizations
☐ Lack of eye contact; head flexion; shoulder flexion
☐ Expressions of shame/guilt
☐ Evaluations of self as unable to deal with events
☐ Rationalizations/rejections of positive feedback
☐ Exaggerations of negative feedback about self
☐ Hesitation to try new things/situations
☐ Denial of problems obvious to others
☐ Projection of blame/responsibility for problems
☐ Rationalization of personal failures
☐ Hypersensitivity to a slight or to a criticism
☐ Grandiosity

ETIOLOGICAL OR RELATED FACTORS
☐ (To be identified)

NOTES

Chronic Low Self-Esteem

DEFINITION

☐ Long-standing negative self-evaluation/feelings about self or self-capabilities which may be directly or indirectly expressed

DEFINING CHARACTERISTICS

☐ Long-standing/chronic:
    Self-negating verbalizations
    Lack of eye contact; head flexion; shoulder flexion
    Expressions of shame/guilt
    Evaluations of self as unable to deal with events
    Rationalizations/rejections of positive feedback
    Exaggerations of negative feedback about self
    Hesitation to try new things/situations
☐ Frequent lack of success in work or other life events
☐ Overly conforming; dependent on others' opinions
☐ Nonassertive/passive
☐ Indecisive
☐ Excessively seeking reassurance

ETIOLOGICAL OR RELATED FACTORS

☐ (To be determined)

NOTES

Situational Low Self-Esteem

DEFINITION
☐ Negative self-evaluation/feelings about self or self-capabilities in response to a loss or change (previous self-evaluation was positive)

DEFINING CHARACTERISTICS
☐ Episodic occurrence of negative self-appraisal in response to life events (e.g., loss, change) in a person with a previous positive self-evaluation
☐ Self-negating verbalizations (e.g., helplessness, uselessness)
☐ Lack of eye contact; head flexion, shoulder flexion
☐ Expressions of shame/guilt
☐ Evaluations of self as unable to handle situations/events
☐ Difficulty in making decisions

ETIOLOGICAL OR RELATED FACTORS
☐ (To be determined)

NOTES

Body Image Disturbance

DEFINITION
☐ Negative feelings or perceptions about characteristics, functions, or limits of body or body part

DEFINING CHARACTERISTICS
☐ *Verbalized actual or perceived change in structure and/or function of body or body part
☐ Verbalized change in lifestyle because of negative feelings or perceptions of body
☐ Verbalized fear of rejection or reaction by others
☐ Repeated verbalizations focusing on past strength, function, or appearance
☐ Verbalized negative feelings about body (dirty, big, small, unsightly)
☐ Verbalized feelings of helplessness, hopelessness, powerlessness in relation to body
☐ Preoccupation with change in body or loss of part
☐ Personalization of part, or loss, by name
☐ Depersonalization of part or loss by impersonal pronoun
☐ Extension of body boundary to incorporate environmental objects (e.g., machines, oxygen, respirator)
☐ Refusal to verify actual change in body or body part
☐ Guilt, shame
☐ Emphasis on remaining strengths or heightened achievement
☐ Repeated expressions of negative feeling about loss of body fluids, addition of body fluids or machines
☐ Change in ability to estimate spatial relationship of body to environment

(Continued)

NOTES

Body Image Disturbance *Continued*

- ☐ Trauma to nonfunctioning part (intentional or nonintentional)
- ☐ Change in social involvement or social relationships
- ☐ Hiding or overexposing body part
- ☐ Not touching body part
- ☐ Not looking at body part
- ☐ Missing body part
- ☐ Actual change in structure and/or function of body or body part

ETIOLOGICAL OR RELATED FACTORS

- ☐ Nonintegration of change (in body characteristics, function, or limits)
- ☐ Perceived developmental imperfections

NOTES

High Risk for Self-Mutilation

DEFINITION

☐ Presence of risk factors for performing an act on the self to injure, but not kill, which produces tissue damage and tension relief

RISK FACTORS

☐ Inability to cope with increased psychological/physiological tension in a healthy manner
☐ Feelings of depression, rejection, self-hatred, separation anxiety, guilt, and depersonalization
☐ Fluctuating emotions
☐ Command hallucinations
☐ Need for sensory stimuli
☐ Parental emotional deprivation
☐ Dysfunctional family

Groups at Risk

☐ Borderline personality disorder, especially females who are 16 to 25 years of age
☐ Psychotic state—frequently males in young adulthood
☐ Emotionally disturbed and/or battered children
☐ Mentally retarded and autistic children
☐ History of self-injury
☐ History of physical, emotional, or sexual abuse

NOTES

Personal Identity Disturbance

DEFINITION

☐ Inability to distinguish between self and nonself

DEFINING CHARACTERISTICS

☐ Inability to distinguish self from others or objects
☐ Verbalizations of ''not knowing who I am''

ETIOLOGICAL OR RELATED FACTORS

☐ (To be determined)

NOTES

ROLE-RELATIONSHIP
PATTERN

NOTES

Anticipatory Grieving

DEFINITION
☐ Expectation of disruption in familiar pattern or significant relationships (includes people, possessions, job, status, home, ideals, parts and processes of the body)

DEFINING CHARACTERISTICS
☐ Potential loss of significant object
☐ Verbal expression of distress at potential (anticipated) loss
☐ Anger
☐ Sadness, sorrow, crying
☐ Crying at frequent intervals, choked feeling
☐ Change in eating habits
☐ Alteration in sleep or dream patterns
☐ Alteration in activity level
☐ Altered libido
☐ Idealization of anticipated loss
☐ Developmental regression
☐ Alterations in concentration or pursuit of tasks

ETIOLOGICAL OR RELATED FACTORS
☐ Expected loss/change (specify)

NOTES

Dysfunctional Grieving

DEFINITION

☐ Extended length (unresolved grieving) or severity of grieving process related to an actual or perceived loss or change in pattern of relationships (includes people, possessions, job, status, home, ideals, parts and processes of the body, etc.)

DEFINING CHARACTERISTICS

☐ Verbal expression of distress at loss or denial of loss
☐ Expression of guilt
☐ Expression of unresolved issues
☐ Anger
☐ Sadness
☐ Crying
☐ Difficulty in expressing meaning of loss
☐ Alterations in eating habits
☐ Alterations of sleep or dream pattern
☐ Alterations in activity level, work, or socialization
☐ Altered libido
☐ Idealization of lost object
☐ Reliving past experiences
☐ Interference with life functioning
☐ Developmental regression
☐ Labile effect
☐ Alterations in concentration and/or pursuits of tasks
☐ Continued indicators of grieving beyond expected time for cultural group

NOTES

Dysfunctional Grieving *Continued*

ETIOLOGICAL OR RELATED FACTORS

- ☐ Loss or perceived loss/change (specify)
- ☐ Unavailable support systems

NOTES

Disturbance in Role Performance

DEFINITION
☐ Change, conflict, denial of role responsibilities or inability to perform role responsibilities

DEFINING CHARACTERISTICS
☐ Denial of role
☐ Conflict in roles
☐ Change in self-perception of role
☐ Change in others' perception of role
☐ Change in physical capacity to resume role
☐ Lack of knowledge of role
☐ Change in usual patterns of responsibilities

ETIOLOGICAL OR RELATED FACTORS
☐ (To be determined)

NOTES

Unresolved Independence-Dependence Conflict

DEFINITION

☐ Lack of resolution of need and desire to be dependent/independent with expectation (therapeutic, maturational, or social) to be independent/dependent

DEFINING CHARACTERISTICS

☐ Repeated verbal expressions of desire for independence (in situations that require some dependence: therapeutic, maturational, or social) or
☐ Repeated verbal expressions of desire for dependence (in situations that require independence (therapeutic, maturational, or social)
☐ Expression of anger
☐ Anxiety

ETIOLOGICAL OR RELATED FACTORS

☐ Physical activity restrictions

NOTES

Social Isolation

DEFINITION

- Interpersonal interaction below level desired or required for personal integrity

DEFINING CHARACTERISTICS

- Apathy
- Verbalization of isolation from others
- Low contact with peers
- Absent or limited contact with community
- Lack of contact with or absence of significant others
- Seclusion

ETIOLOGICAL OR RELATED FACTORS

- Impaired mobility
- Therapeutic isolation
- Sociocultural dissonance
- Insufficient community resources
- Body image disturbance
- Fear (environmental hazards, violence)

NOTES

Social Isolation *or Social Rejection*

DEFINITION
- Condition of aloneness experienced by the individual and perceived as imposed by others and as a negative or threatening state

DEFINING CHARACTERISTICS
- Expresses feelings of aloneness imposed by others, rejection, or feelings of difference from others
- Expresses values acceptable to subculture but unacceptable to dominant cultural group
- Perceived inadequacy of significant purpose in life or absence of purpose in life
- Perceived inability to meet expectations of others or insecurity in public
- Observed or expressed interests/activities inappropriate to the developmental age/stage
- Shows behavior unaccepted by dominant cultural group
- Seeks to be alone or to exist in a subculture
- Sad, dull affect
- Uncommunicative, withdrawn, no eye contact
- Projects hostility in voice, behavior
- Preoccupation with own thoughts, repetitive meaningless actions
- Absence of supportive significant other(s): family, friends, group

ETIOLOGICAL OR RELATED FACTORS
- Alteration in physical appearance or mental status
- Developmental delay
- Immature interests
- Unacceptable social behavior or values
- Altered state of wellness
- Inability to engage in satisfying personal relationships

NOTES

Impaired Social Interaction

DEFINITION

- □ The state in which an individual participates in an insufficient or excessive quantity or ineffective quality of social exchange

DEFINING CHARACTERISTICS

- □ *Verbalized or observed discomfort in social situations
- □ *Verbalized or observed inability to receive or communicate a satisfying sense of belonging, caring, interest, or shared history
- □ *Observed use of unsuccessful social interaction behaviors
- □ *Dysfunctional interaction with peers, family, and/or others
- □ Family report of change of style or patterns of interaction

ETIOLOGICAL OR RELATED FACTORS

- □ Knowledge/skill deficit (ways to enhance mutuality)
- □ Communication barriers
- □ Self-concept disturbance
- □ Absence of available significant others/peers
- □ Limited physical mobility
- □ Therapeutic isolation
- □ Sociocultural dissonance
- □ Environmental barriers
- □ Altered thought processes

NOTES

Altered Growth and Development: Social Skills (Specify)[1]

DEFINITION

☐ Demonstrates deviations from age-group norms in acquisition of social skills

DEFINING CHARACTERISTICS

☐ *Delay or difficulty in acquisition of social interaction skills typical of age group/developmental level
☐ Dysfunctional interactions

ETIOLOGICAL OR RELATED FACTORS

☐ Environmental/stimulation/modeling deficiencies
☐ Inconsistent responsiveness
☐ Multiple caretakers, inadequate caretaking
☐ Separation (from significant others)
☐ Physical disability effects
☐ Indifference
☐ Self-esteem disturbance
☐ Social isolation

[1]See p. 215, Altered Growth and Development, for accepted diagnosis.

NOTES

Relocation Stress Syndrome *or* *Relocation Syndrome*

DEFINITION

- ☐ Physiological and/or psychosocial disturbances as a result of transfer from one environment to another

DEFINING CHARACTERISTICS

- ☐ *Change in environment/location
- ☐ *Anxiety, apprehension
- ☐ *Depression, sad affect
- ☐ *Increased confusion (elderly population)
- ☐ *Expressions of loneliness
- ☐ Moderate to high degree of environment change†
- ☐ Verbalization of being concerned/upset about transfer
- ☐ Verbalization of unwillingness to relocate
- ☐ Unfavorable comparison of post- with pretransfer staff
- ☐ Little or no preparation for impending move†
- ☐ History of previous transfers (same/different type)†
- ☐ Losses involved with decision to move†
- ☐ Concurrent/recent/past losses†
- ☐ Feeling of powerlessness regarding move†
- ☐ Dependency
- ☐ Insecurity, lack of trust
- ☐ Support system deficit†
- ☐ Restlessness, vigilance, or withdrawal
- ☐ Sleep pattern disturbance
- ☐ Change in eating habits, gastrointestinal disturbances
- ☐ Weight change
- ☐ Impaired health status (psychosocial/physical)†

†Replaces the nonapproved diagnosis, Translocation Syndrome. Generally, the probable cause of a syndrome is contained in the name (e.g., relocation). Related factors were approved by NANDA for this syndrome.

NOTES

Altered Family Processes

DEFINITION
☐ Inability of family system (household members) to meet needs of members, carry out family functions, or maintain communications for mutual growth and maturation.

DEFINING CHARACTERISTICS
☐ Inability of family members to relate to each other for mutual growth and maturation
☐ Failure to send and receive clear messages
☐ Poorly communicated family rules, rituals, symbols; unexamined myths
☐ Unhealthy family decision-making processes
☐ Inability of family members to express and accept wide range of feelings
☐ Inability to accept and receive help
☐ Does not demonstrate respect for individuality and autonomy of members
☐ Rigidity in functions and roles
☐ Fails to accomplish current (or past) family developmental tasks
☐ Inappropriate (nonproductive) boundary maintenance
☐ Inability to adapt to change
☐ Inability to deal with traumatic or crisis experience constructively
☐ Parents do not demonstrate respect for each other's views on child-rearing practices
☐ Inappropriate (nonproductive) level and direction of energy
☐ Inability to meet needs of members (physical, security, emotional, spiritual)
☐ Family uninvolved in community activities

(Continued)

NOTES

Altered Family Processes *Continued*

ETIOLOGICAL OR RELATED FACTORS

- ☐ Situational crisis or transition
- ☐ Developmental crisis or transition

NOTES

High Risk for Altered Parenting

DEFINITION

☐ Presence of risk factors during prenatal or child-rearing period that may interfere with process of adjustment to parenting

DEFINING CHARACTERISTICS (RISK FACTORS)

☐ Unavailable or ineffective role model
☐ History of physical and psychosocial abuse (of nurturing figure)
☐ Support system deficit (between/from significant others)
☐ Unmet social, emotional, developmental needs (of parenting figures)
☐ Interruption in bonding process (maternal, paternal, other)
☐ Unrealistic expectation (self, infant, partner)
☐ Perceived threat to own survival (physical, emotional)
☐ Physical impairment (blindness, etc.)
☐ Physical or mental illness
☐ Presence of stress (financial, legal, recent personal crisis, cultural change, multiple pregnancies)
☐ Knowledge or skill deficit (specify: parenting skills, developmental progression, etc.)
☐ Limited cognitive functioning
☐ Lack of role identity
☐ Lack of, or inappropriate, response of child to relationship
☐ Social isolation
☐ Fear (specify focus)

NOTES

Altered Parenting

DEFINITION

☐ Inability of nurturing figure(s) to create an environment which promotes optimum growth and development of another human being (NOTE: Adjustment to parenting, in general, is a normal maturation process following birth of a child.)

DEFINING CHARACTERISTICS

☐ *Inattentive to infant/child needs
☐ *Inappropriate caretaking behaviors, (toilet training, feeding, sleep/rest, etc.)
☐ *History of child abuse or abandonment by primary caretaker
☐ Actual alteration:
    Verbalization cannot control child
    Abandonment of infant/child
    Runaway
    Incidence of physical and psychological trauma
☐ Lack of parental attachment behaviors
☐ Inappropriate visual, tactile, auditory stimulation
☐ Negative identification of infant/child's characteristics
☐ Negative attachment of meanings to infant/child's characteristics; verbalization of resentment toward infant/child
☐ Verbalization cannot control child
☐ Evidence of physical and psychological trauma to infant/child
☐ Constant verbalization of disappointment in gender or physical characteristics of the infant/child
☐ Verbalization of role inadequacy
☐ Verbal disgust at body functions of infant/child
☐ Noncompliance with health appointments for infant/child or self

(Continued)

NOTES

Altered Parenting *Continued*

☐ Inappropriate or inconsistent discipline practices
☐ Frequent accidents (infant/child); frequent illness (infant/child)
☐ Growth and development lag of infant/child
☐ Verbalizes desire to have child call parent by first name versus traditional, cultural tendencies
☐ Child receives care from multiple caretakers without consideration for the needs of the infant/child
☐ Compulsively seeks role approval from others

ETIOLOGICAL OR RELATED FACTORS

☐ Knowledge or skill deficit (specify: parenting skills, developmental guidelines, etc.)
☐ Fear (specify focus)
☐ Social isolation
☐ Physical impairment (blindness, etc.)
☐ Mental or physical illness
☐ Support system deficit (between/from significant other[s])
☐ Interrupted parent-infant bonding (e.g., illness of newborn)
☐ Family or personal stress (financial, legal, recent crisis, cultural change, multiple pregnancies)
☐ Unmet social, emotional, or developmental needs (of parenting figures)
☐ Interruption in bonding process (i.e., maternal, paternal, other)
☐ Unrealistic expectations (self, infant, partner)
☐ Perceived threat to own survival (physical and emotional)
☐ Lack of role identity
☐ Lack of or inappropriate response of child
☐ Physical or psychosocial abuse (of nurturing figure)
☐ Limited cognitive functioning

NOTES

Parental Role Conflict

DEFINITION
- Role confusion and conflict in response to crisis experienced by a parent or parents

DEFINING CHARACTERISTICS
- Expresses concerns/feelings of inadequacy to provide for child's physical and emotional needs during hospitalization or in the home
- Expresses concerns about changes in parental role, family functioning, family communication, family health
- Demonstrates disruption in caretaking routines
- Expresses concern about perceived loss of control over decisions relating to child
- Is reluctant to participate in usual caretaking activities, even with encouragement and support
- Verbalizes/demonstrates feelings of guilt, anger, fear, anxiety, and/or frustrations about effect of child's illness on family process

ETIOLOGICAL OR RELATED FACTORS
- Parent-child separation (due to chronic illness)
- Intimidation with invasive or restrictive modalities (e.g., isolation, intubation, specialized-care centers, policies)
- Home care of a child with special needs (e.g., apnea monitoring, postural drainage, hyperalimentation)
- Change in marital status
- Interruptions in family life due to home-care regimen (treatments, caregivers, lack of respite)

NOTES

Parent-Infant Separation

DEFINITION

- Presence of factors that prohibit interaction between infant and parent(s)

DEFINING CHARACTERISTICS

- *Infrequent contact with infant
- Inability of parent(s) to visit hospital regularly
- Absent or limited opportunity for eye-to-eye contact between infant and parent(s)
- Absent or limited opportunity for tactile interaction
- Inability of infant to tolerate noise/touch
- Lack of immediate access to infant
- Verbalization by parent(s) indicating fear of interaction (e.g., fear that infant may die, fear of hurting infant)
- Verbalization by parent(s) regarding inability to parent the infant because of separation/lack of knowledge about the infant
- Lack of immediate information regarding infant's condition

ETIOLOGICAL OR RELATED FACTORS

- Prematurity
- Critical illness of infant or parent(s)
- Hospitalization of infant or parent(s)
- Transportation difficulties for family to visit hospitalized infant
- Support system deficit (e.g., lack of care relief to enable visitation)

NOTES

Weak Mother-Infant Attachment *or* Parent-Infant Attachment

DEFINITION

☐ Pattern of unreciprocal bonding relationship between parent and infant or primary caretaker and infant

DEFINING CHARACTERISTICS

☐ Minimal smiling, close contact, enfolding, talking to baby
☐ Does not assume "en-face" position, eye-to-eye contact
☐ Minimal touching, stroking, patting, rocking, holding, kissing of infant except when necessary to feed or change diapers
☐ Does not attempt comforting responses to crying or continues unsuccessful methods
☐ Low reciprocal interaction pattern (e.g., minimal smiling, babbling response to touching, kissing, etc.)
☐ Irritable infant or low responsiveness to parent
☐ Few positive comments about infant; expressions of disappointment
☐ Bottle propped or tense posture during breast feeding
☐ Infrequent visitation of hospitalized infant (e.g., less than twice a week)
☐ Prenatal history of ambivalence, negative feelings regarding pregnancy
☐ High-risk adolescent parent, physically or mentally ill parent

(Continued)

Weak Mother-Infant Attachment *or* Parent-Infant Attachment *Continued*

ETIOLOGICAL OR RELATED FACTORS

- ☐ Parental anxiety
- ☐ Fear (specify)
- ☐ Parent-infant separation
- ☐ Perceived low parenting competency (infant care)
- ☐ Low (infant) social responsiveness
- ☐ Support system deficit
- ☐ Family stress

NOTES

Caregiver Role Strain

DEFINITION
☐ Caregiver perceives difficulty in performing the family caregiver role

DEFINING CHARACTERISTICS
Caregiver's report:
☐ Inadequate resources to provide required care
☐ Difficulty providing specific caregiving activities
☐ Worry about the care receiver (e.g., care receiver's health
and emotional state, having to put the care receiver in an in-
stitution, and/or who will care for the care receiver if some-
thing should happen to the caregiver)
☐ Feeling that caregiving interferes with other important roles
in caregiver's life
☐ Feeling of loss because the care receiver is "like a different
person" compared with before caregiving began
☐ In the case of a child, feeling of loss that the care receiver
was not the child the caregiver expected
☐ Family conflict around issues of providing care
☐ Stress or nervousness in caregiver's relationship with the care
receiver
☐ Depression

ETIOLOGICAL OR RELATED FACTORS
Pathophysiological/Physiological
☐ Illness severity; unpredictable course of illness; unstable
health (care receiver)
☐ Caregiver health impairment
☐ Addiction/codependency
☐ Premature birth/congenital defect   *(Continued)*

NOTES

Caregiver Role Strain *Continued*

- ☐ Discharge of family member with significant home care needs
- ☐ Caregiver is female

Developmental

- ☐ Caregiver not developmentally ready for caregiver role (e.g., young adult needing to provide care for a middle-aged parent)
- ☐ Developmental delay/retardation (care receiver or caregiver)

Psychosocial

- ☐ Psychological or cognitive problems (care receiver)
- ☐ Deviant/bizarre behavior (care receiver)
- ☐ Marginal family adaptation/dysfunction (before caregiving situation)
- ☐ Marginal coping patterns (caregiver)
- ☐ History of poor relationship (caregiver-care receiver)
- ☐ Caregiver is spouse

Situational

- ☐ Family/caregiver isolation
- ☐ Presence of abuse or violence
- ☐ Situational family stressors (e.g., significant loss; disaster/crisis; poverty/economic vulnerability; major life events: birth, death, hospitalization, leaving/returning home, marriage, divorce, employment changes, retirement)
- ☐ Duration of caregiving
- ☐ Inadequate physical environment for providing care (e.g., housing, transportation, community services, equipment)
- ☐ Lack of respite/recreation (caregiver)
- ☐ Inexperience with caregiving
- ☐ Competing role commitments (caregiver)
- ☐ Complexity/amount of caregiving tasks

NOTES

High Risk for Caregiver Role Strain

DEFINITION
☐ Caregiver is vulnerable for perceived difficulty in performing the family caregiver role

RISK FACTORS
Pathophysiological
☐ Illness severity; unpredictable course of illness; unstable health (care receiver)
☐ Caregiver health impairment
☐ Addiction/codependency
☐ Premature birth/congenital defect
☐ Discharge of family member with significant home care needs
☐ Caregiver is female

Developmental
☐ Caregiver not developmentally ready for caregiver role (e.g., young adult needing to provide care for middle-aged parent)
☐ Developmental delay/retardation (care receiver or caregiver)

Psychological
☐ Psychological or cognitive problems (care receiver)
☐ Marginal family adaptation/dysfunction (before the caregiving situation)
☐ Marginal coping patterns (caregiver)
☐ History of poor relationship (caregiver-care receiver)
☐ Caregiver is spouse
☐ Deviant/bizarre behavior (care receiver)   *(Continued)*

NOTES

High Risk for Caregiver Role
Strain *Continued*

Situational

☐ Family/caregiver isolation

☐ Presence of abuse or violence

☐ Situational family stressors (specify, e.g., significant loss; disaster/crisis; poverty/economic vulnerability; major life events: birth, death, hospitalization, leaving/returning home, marriage, divorce, employment changes, retirement)

☐ Duration of caregiving

☐ Inadequate physical environment for providing care (e.g., housing, transportation, community services, equipment)

☐ Lack of respite/recreation (caregiver)

☐ Inexperience with caregiving

☐ Competing role commitments (caregiver)

☐ Complexity/amount of caregiving tasks

NOTES

Impaired Verbal Communication

DEFINITION
- Reduced, or absent, ability to use language in human interaction

DEFINING CHARACTERISTICS
- *Unable to speak dominant language
- *Speaks or verbalizes with difficulty
- *Does not, or cannot, speak
- Stuttering
- Slurring
- Difficulty forming words or sentences
- Difficulty expressing thought verbally
- Inappropriate verbalization
- Dyspnea
- Disorientation

ETIOLOGICAL OR RELATED FACTORS
- Decrease in circulation to brain
- Anatomical defects (cleft palate)
- Cultural difference
- Physical barrier (brain tumor, tracheostomy, intubation)
- Psychological barrier (psychosis, lack of stimuli)
- Developmental or age-related

NOTES

Altered Growth and Development: Communication Skills (Specify)[1]

DEFINITION

- Demonstrates deviations from age-group norms in development of communication skills

DEFINING CHARACTERISTICS

- *Delay or difficulty in performing expressive, communication skills typical of age group/developmental level (prelanguage vocalization, language skills, signs, etc.)
- Flat affect
- Listlessness
- Decreased responses

ETIOLOGICAL OR RELATED FACTORS

- Environmental/stimulation deficiencies
- Inconsistent responsiveness
- Multiple caregivers, inadequate caregiving
- Separation (from significant others)
- Physical disability effects
- Prescribed dependence
- Indifference

[1]See p. 215 Altered Growth and Development, for accepted diagnosis.

NOTES

High Risk for Violence

DEFINITION
☐ Presence of risk factors for self-directed or other-directed physical trauma

DEFINING CHARACTERISTICS (RISK FACTORS)
☐ *Angry facial expressions
☐ *Rigid posture; clenched fists
☐ *Tautness indicating intense effort for self-control
☐ *Increased motor activity, pacing, excitement, irritability, agitation
☐ *Hostile threatening verbalizations
☐ *Boasting prior abuse of others or history of prior abuse of others
☐ *Overt and aggressive acts: Goal-directed destruction of objects in environment
☐ *Possession of destructive means (gun, knife, weapon, etc.)
☐ *Rage
☐ *Self-destructive behavior (active, aggressive or suicidal acts)
☐ *Substance abuse or withdrawal
☐ *Suspicion of others (paranoid ideation, delusions, hallucinations)
☐ Increasing anxiety level
☐ Fear of self or others
☐ Inability to verbalize feelings
☐ High situational stress factors
☐ Antisocial character disturbance
☐ Catatonic or manic excitement
☐ Organic brain syndrome
☐ Rage reactions, child abuse   (*Continued*)

NOTES

Potential for Violence *Continued*

- ☐ Temporal lobe epilepsy
- ☐ Anger
- ☐ Repeated complaints, requests, and demands
- ☐ Provocative acts (argumentation, hypersensitivity, overreaction, dissatisfaction)
- ☐ Depression (active, aggressive, suicidal acts)
- ☐ Vulnerable self-esteem

NOTES

SEXUALITY-REPRODUCTIVE PATTERN

NOTES

Sexual Dysfunction

DEFINITION

☐ Perceived problem in achieving desired satisfaction of sexuality

DEFINING CHARACTERISTICS

☐ Verbalizations of problem in sexuality
☐ Alterations in achieving perceived sex role
☐ Actual or perceived limitation imposed by disease and/or therapy
☐ Conflicts involving values
☐ Alteration in achieving sexual satisfaction
☐ Inability to achieve desired sexual satisfaction
☐ Frequent seeking of confirmation of desirability
☐ Alteration in relationship with significant other
☐ Change of interest in self and others

ETIOLOGICAL OR RELATED FACTORS

☐ Ineffectual or absent models
☐ Physical abuse
☐ Psychosocial abuse (e.g., harmful relationships)
☐ Vulnerability
☐ Misinformation or lack of knowledge
☐ Values conflict
☐ Lack of privacy
☐ Lack of significant other
☐ Altered body structure or function (pregnancy, recent childbirth, drugs, surgery, anomalies, disease process, trauma, radiation)

NOTES

Altered Sexuality Patterns

DEFINITION
☐ The state in which an individual expresses concern regarding his/her sexuality

DEFINING CHARACTERISTICS
☐ *Reported difficulties, limitations, or changes in sexual behaviors or activities

ETIOLOGICAL OR RELATED FACTORS
☐ Knowledge/skill deficit (alternative responses to health-related transitions)
☐ Altered body function/structure
☐ Illness or medical treatment
☐ Lack of privacy
☐ Lack of significant other
☐ Ineffective or absent role models
☐ Conflicts with sexual orientation or variant preferences
☐ Fear (pregnancy)
☐ Fear (acquiring sexually transmitted disease)
☐ Impaired relationship with significant other

NOTES

Rape Trauma Syndrome

DEFINITION

☐ Forced, violent sexual penetration against victim's will and without victim's consent (syndrome includes an acute phase of disorganization of victim's lifestyle and a long-term process of reorganization of lifestyle).

DEFINING CHARACTERISTICS
Acute Phase

☐ Report of forced, violent, sexual penetration
☐ Anger
☐ Embarrassment
☐ Fear of physical violence and death
☐ Humiliation
☐ Revenge
☐ Self-blame
☐ Multiple physical symptoms (e.g., gastro-intestinal irritability, genito-urinary discomfort, increased muscle tension, sleep-pattern disturbance)

Long-Term Phase

☐ Changes in lifestyle (changes in residence, dealing with repetitive nightmares and phobias, seeking social network support)

NOTES

Rape Trauma Syndrome: Compound Reaction

DEFINITION
☐ Victim experiences symptoms described for rape trauma (physical or psychiatric illness, reliance on alcohol or drugs)

DEFINING CHARACTERISTICS
☐ See defining characteristics listed under Rape Trauma Syndrome
☐ Reactivated symptoms of previous conditions (i.e., physical illness, psychiatric illness)
☐ Reliance on alcohol and/or drugs

NOTES

Rape Trauma Syndrome: Silent Reaction

DEFINITION
☐ Presence of signs and symptoms but without victim's mentioning to anyone that rape has occurred

DEFINING CHARACTERISTICS
☐ See defining characteristics listed under Rape Trauma Syndrome; no initial verbalization of the occurrence of rape
☐ Abrupt changes in relationships with men
☐ Increase in nightmares
☐ Increasing anxiety during interview (blocking of associations, long periods of silence, minor stuttering, physical distress)
☐ Marked changes in sexual behavior with opposite sex
☐ Sudden onset of phobic reactions

NOTES

COPING–STRESS-TOLERANCE
PATTERN

NOTES

Ineffective Coping (Individual)

DEFINITION
☐ Impairment of adaptive behaviors and problem-solving abilities for meeting life's demands and roles. (Methods of handling stressful life situations are insufficient to control anxiety, fear, or anger.)

DEFINING CHARACTERISTICS
☐ *Verbalization of inability to cope
☐ *Inability to ask for help
☐ Inability to solve problem effectively
☐ Anxiety, fear, anger, irritability, tension
☐ Presence of life stress
☐ Inability to meet role expectations
☐ Inability to meet basic needs
☐ Alteration in societal participation
☐ Destructive behavior toward self and others
☐ Inappropriate or ineffective use of defense mechanisms
☐ Change in usual communication patterns
☐ High rate of accidents
☐ Verbal manipulation
☐ Excess food intake, alcohol consumption; smoking
☐ Digestive, bowel, appetite disturbance; chronic fatigue or sleep pattern disturbance

ETIOLOGICAL OR RELATED FACTORS
☐ Situational crises (specify type)
☐ Maturational crises (specify type)
☐ Personal vulnerability
☐ Knowledge deficit (specify)
☐ Problem-solving skills deficit

NOTES

Avoidance Coping[1]

DEFINITION

- [ ] Prolonged minimization or denial of information (facts, meanings, consequences) when a situation requires active coping

DEFINING CHARACTERISTICS

- [ ] Presence of perceived threat to health, self-image, values, lifestyle, or relationships
- [ ] Minimizes, ignores, or forgets information following clear communication or observation
- [ ] Mislabeling of events
- [ ] Absence of problem solving, information seeking, incorporation of new information into future planning
- [ ] Regressive dependency
- [ ] Anxiety, depression, passivity, or anger

ETIOLOGICAL OR RELATED FACTORS

- [ ] Perceived incompetency
- [ ] Perceived powerlessness
- [ ] Support system deficit
- [ ] Independence-dependence conflict (adolescent)

[1]Avoidance or denial is a constructive response to events or consequences when ambiguity or doubt exists. Avoidance is not to be confused with hope or adaptive denial.

NOTES

Defensive Coping

DEFINITION
☐ Repeated projection of falsely positive self-evaluation based on a self-protective pattern which defends against underlying perceived threats to positive self-regard

DEFINING CHARACTERISTICS
☐ Denial of obvious problems/weaknesses
☐ Projection of blame/responsibility
☐ Rationalization of failures
☐ Hypersensitivity to a slight or to a criticism
☐ Grandiosity
☐ Superior attitude toward others
☐ Difficulty establishing/maintaining relationships
☐ Hostile laughter or ridicule of others
☐ Difficulty in reality testing of perceptions
☐ Lack of follow-through or participation in treatment or therapy

ETIOLOGICAL OR RELATED FACTORS
☐ Perceived threat to self (specify)

NOTES

Ineffective Denial *or Denial*[1]

DEFINITION

☐ Conscious or unconscious attempt to disavow the knowledge/ meaning of an event to reduce anxiety/fear (to the detriment of health)

DEFINING CHARACTERISTICS

☐ Delays seeking/refuses health care attention to the detriment of health
☐ Does not perceive personal relevance of symptoms or danger
☐ Uses home remedies (e.g., self-treatment) to relieve symptoms
☐ Does not admit fear of death or invalidism; displaces fear of impact of the condition
☐ Minimizes symptoms; displaces source of symptoms to other organs
☐ Displays inappropriate affect
☐ Is unable to admit impact of disease on life pattern
☐ Makes dismissive gestures or comments when speaking of distressing events

ETIOLOGICAL OR RELATED FACTORS

☐ Perceived threat to self (specify)

---

[1]It is unclear whether the adjective *ineffective* before the word *denial* relates to the diagnosis, its etiology, or its consequences. It is not consistent with definition and characteristics specified. *Suggestion:* Use *Denial* or see *Avoidance Coping* (p. 357).

NOTES

Impaired Adjustment

DEFINITION

☐ The state in which the individual is unable to modify his/her life-style/behavior in a manner consistent with a change in health status

DEFINING CHARACTERISTICS

☐ *Verbalization of nonacceptance of health status change
☐ *Nonexistent or unsuccessful ability to be involved in problem solving or goal setting
☐ Lack of movement toward independence
☐ Extended period of shock, disbelief, or anger regarding health status change
☐ Lack of future-oriented thinking

ETIOLOGICAL OR RELATED FACTORS

☐ Inadequate support system
☐ Sensory overload
☐ Assault to self-esteem
☐ Altered locus of control
☐ Incomplete grieving
☐ Disability requiring lifestyle change
☐ Impaired cognition

NOTES

Post-Trauma Response

DEFINITION

☐ The state of an individual experiencing a sustained painful response to an unexpected extraordinary life event(s)

DEFINING CHARACTERISTICS

☐ *Reexperience of the traumatic event which may be identified in cognitive, affective, and/or sensory-motor activities:
   Flashbacks
   Intrusive thoughts
   Repetitive dreams or nightmares
   Excessive verbalization of the traumatic event
   Verbalization of survival guilt or
   Guilt about behavior required for survival
☐ Psychic/emotional numbness:
   Impaired interpretation of reality
   Confusion
   Dissociation or
   Amnesia
   Vagueness about traumatic event
   Constricted affect
☐ Altered lifestyle:
   Self-destructiveness, such as substance abuse, suicide attempt, or other acting-out behavior
   Difficulty with interpersonal relationships
   Development of phobia regarding the trauma
   Poor impulse control/irritability and explosiveness

(Continued)

NOTES

Post-Trauma Response *Continued*

ETIOLOGICAL OR RELATED FACTORS

☐ Disasters
☐ Wars
☐ Epidemics
☐ Rape
☐ Assault
☐ Torture
☐ Catastrophic illness or accident

NOTES

Family Coping: Potential for Growth

DEFINITION
☐ Family member has effectively managed adaptive tasks involved with the client's health challenge and is exhibiting desire and readiness for enhanced health and growth in regard to self and in relation to the client

DEFINING CHARACTERISTICS
☐ Family member attempts to describe growth impact of crisis on his or her own values, priorities, goals, or relationships
☐ Family member is moving in direction of health-promoting and enriching lifestyle which supports and monitors maturational processes, audits and negotiates treatment programs, and generally chooses experiences which optimize wellness
☐ Individual expresses interest in making contact on a one-to-one basis or on a mutual-aid group basis with another person who has experienced a similar situation

ETIOLOGICAL OR RELATED FACTORS (factor is summarized)
☐ Readiness for seeking self-actualization

NOTES

Ineffective Family Coping: Compromised

DEFINITION
☐ Usually supportive primary person (family member or close friend) providing insufficient, ineffective, or compromised support, comfort, assistance, or encouragement which may be needed by client to manage or master adaptive tasks related to health challenge

DEFINING CHARACTERISTICS
☐ Client expresses concern or complaint about significant other's response to his/her health problem
☐ Significant person describes preoccupation with personal reactions (e.g., fear, guilt, anticipatory grief, anxiety) to client's illness, disability, or other situational or developmental crises
☐ Significant person describes or confirms inadequate understanding of knowledge base which interferes with effective assistive or supportive behaviors
☐ Significant person attempts assistive or supportive behaviors with less than satisfactory results
☐ Significant person withdraws or enters into limited or temporary personal communication with client at time of need
☐ Significant person displays protective behavior disproportionate (too little or too much) to client's abilities or need for autonomy

ETIOLOGICAL OR RELATED FACTORS (factors are summarized)
☐ Knowledge deficit
☐ Emotional conflicts
☐ Exhaustion of supportive capacity   *(Continued)*

NOTES

Ineffective Family Coping: Compromised

Continued

☐ Role changes (family)
☐ Temporary family disorganization
☐ Developmental or situational crises

NOTES

Ineffective Family Coping: Disabling

DEFINITION

☐ Behavior of significant person (family member or primary person) disables own capacities and client's capacities to effectively address tasks essential to either person's adaptation to the health challenge

DEFINING CHARACTERISTICS

☐ Neglectful care of client in regard to basic human needs and/or illness treatment
☐ Distortion of reality regarding client's health problem including extreme denial about existence or severity
☐ Intolerance
☐ Rejection
☐ Abandonment
☐ Desertion
☐ Carrying on usual routines disregarding client's needs
☐ Psychosomaticism
☐ Taking on illness signs of the client
☐ Decisions and actions by family which are detrimental to economic or social well-being
☐ Agitation, depression, aggression, hostility
☐ Impaired restructuring of a meaningful life for self, impaired individuation, prolonged overconcern for client
☐ Neglectful relationships with other family members
☐ Client's development of helpless, inactive dependence

(Continued)

NOTES

Ineffective Family Coping: Disabling

Continued

ETIOLOGICAL OR RELATED FACTORS
☐ Chronically unexpressed guilt/anxiety/hostility/etc. (significant other)
☐ Dissonant discrepancy of coping styles (for dealing with adaptive tasks by the significant person and client or among significant people)
☐ Highly ambivalent family relationships
☐ Arbitrary handling of family's resistance to treatment (which tends to solidify defensiveness as it fails to deal adequately with underlying anxiety)

NOTES

VALUE-BELIEF PATTERN

NOTES

Spiritual Distress (Distress of Human Spirit)

DEFINITION

☐ A disruption in the life principle which pervades a person's entire being and which integrates and transcends biopsychosocial nature

DEFINING CHARACTERISTICS

☐ *Expressed concern with meaning of life/death and/or belief system
☐ Anger toward God
☐ Questions meaning of suffering
☐ Verbalizes inner conflict about beliefs
☐ Verbalizes concern about relationship with deity
☐ Questions meaning for own existence
☐ Unable to participate in usual religious practices
☐ Seeks spiritual assistance
☐ Questions moral/ethical implications of therapeutic regime
☐ Gallows humor
☐ Displacement of anger toward religious representatives
☐ Description of nightmares/sleep disturbance
☐ Alteration in behavior/mood evidenced by anger, crying, withdrawal, preoccupation, anxiety, hostility, apathy, etc.

ETIOLOGY

☐ Separation from religious/cultural ties
☐ Challenged belief and value system (e.g., due to moral/ethical implications of therapy, intense suffering, etc.)

NOTES

Index